Mindful Life Weight Loss

Mindful Eating — Holistic, Sustainable Weight Loss

Mindful Life Weight Loss

Mindful Life Weight Loss

Mindful Eating — Holistic, Sustainable Weight Loss

Kim Gold, MS, RYT

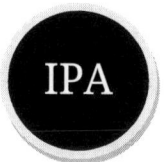

Integrated Peace Arts Press
Scarsdale, NY

Mindful Life Weight Loss

Mindful Life Weight Loss: Mindful Eating – Holistic, Sustainable Weight Loss

Kim Gold, MS, RYT

Copyright © 2015 Kim Gold

All rights reserved.

ISBN-13: 978-1515372639
ISBN-10: 1515372634

Publisher's Note: This book is written as a source of information only. The information contained in this book should by no means be considered a substitute for the advice of a qualified medical professional, who should always be consulted before beginning any new diet, exercise, or other health program.

All efforts have been made to ensure the accuracy of the information contained in this book as of the date published. The authors expressly disclaim responsibility for any adverse effects arising from the use or application of the information contained herein. All names and identifying details have been changed in the Mindful Life in Action sections.

Mindful Life Weight Loss

DEDICATION
This book is dedicated to my two wonderful daughters—the lights of my life.

Mindful Life Weight Loss

Mindful Life Weight Loss

CONTENTS

Acknowledgments

Introduction   11

1 Start From Where You Are   15

2 What is a Mindful Life   29

3 Setting Goals   45

4 Mindfulness and Food   63

5 Mindful Eating   77

6	Born to Move	87
7	Effortless Exercise	97
8	Thinking in Systems	109
9	Gaining Leverage, Increasing Momentum	119
10	Green Time vs. Screen Time	133
11	Beyond Ourselves	143
12	Emotional Eating	155
13	Measuring Success	163
	Conclusion	169

Additional Resources   171

ACKNOWLEDGMENTS

This book would not be possible without the generosity of those who have shared the ancient practice of mindfulness, and continued these teachings for future generations. I express my gratitude to Thich Nhat Hanh and his lineage, and to my teachers and mentors in Eastern and Western wisdom traditions.

Mindful Life Weight Loss

Introduction

> **MINDFULNESS PRACTICES ENHANCE THE CONNECTION BETWEEN OUR BODY, OUR MIND AND EVERYTHING ELSE THAT IS AROUND US. MINDFUL LIVING IS THE KEY TO UNDERSTANDING OUR STRUGGLES WITH WEIGHT AND TO EMPOWERING US TO CONTROL OUR WEIGHT.**
>
> THICH NHAT HANH

Just about everyone is trying to lose weight, keep from gaining weight, or making peace with their body the way it is. For much of my life, I was no exception. Growing up female in America had set me at war with my body, in spite of being a "healthy weight." It hasn't been easy. It wasn't until I reached middle age that I finally felt at peace with my weight. It wasn't my weight that changed. It was my mind.

Things shifted for me when I began to study Zen meditation, particularly mindfulness. Mindfulness showed me how to become a compassionate observer of myself. It helped me to detach from cultural pressures and internalized messages and tune into my body's innate wisdom. I combined training in mindfulness with my academic studies and clinical work in Marriage and Family Therapy (MFT) to create the Mindful Life Weight Loss program. I, along with my partner, Steve Kanney, have been teaching this program to people in our Westchester County, New York locations, as well as online, with great success. I wrote this book to share the program with an even larger audience, and to provide a voice of balance and compassion in the brutal world of diets and weight loss.

If you are beginning this book: welcome to the first step on the path toward ending your battle with weight. Perhaps you have had a lifetime of dieting, and are exhausted by constant vigilance and deprivation. Maybe your weight has gotten to a point where you are afraid to even step on the scale. Or maybe you don't have any more weight to lose, but are concerned that the weight will come back again. Your weight may be considered normal, but you still struggle with unhappiness about your body. It is time to end the struggle, and start on the path of peace.

Wherever you are, regardless of how many times you have tried: that is perfect. It is the beginning. Start from a place of acceptance and compassion, and take one step at a time.

The Mindful Life Weight Loss program is different from many others because it uses the skill of mindfulness to put you in touch with yourself. Mindfulness is compassionate, nonjudgmental awareness of the present moment and your thoughts, feelings, and needs. Mindfulness is what is missing from our fragmented and over-stimulated modern lifestyle. We have become increasingly mindless and removed from what our bodies and minds need. This vacuum is filled with countless voices telling us what we should eat or how we should look. Reconnecting

Mindful Life Weight Loss

with yourself is the most important step you can take. From there, it is your own inner wisdom that will direct you toward your personal version of a Mindful Life. There is no "one size fits all" or big box solution. There is only your solution.

Mindfulness is like a muscle. The more you use it, the stronger it becomes. This book will help you strengthen this muscle through practice, and use it to make changes and achieve goals.

Losing weight--and keeping it off---must be viewed in a holistic context. Every area of a person's life affects the others. The Mindful Life Weight Loss program does not simply look at food, count calories, or prescribe a workout plan. These are band-aids. This program is an integrated system that can help you examine each area of your life--step by step--- and understand how it relates to your weight and overall health.

Use this book as an interactive tool. Take your time with each chapter, allowing its wisdom to take root in your life. You may want to read through the entire book and then go back and do one chapter per week, or one chapter every two weeks. Find a pace that works for you. You will be asked to begin each chapter with a few minutes of mindful silence. Don't skip this part! These brief minutes contain potent seeds of change. You'll see.

As you read this book, make notations of any connections or insights that arise. Use this book as a journal, recording your milestones and struggles. Rather than view your weight as an obstacle, think of it as your entry point into healing. To that end, it is helpful to designate a "sacred space" for your work. Set aside an area of your home, and find some way to set it apart from the ordinary. A vase of flowers, a candle, a plant, or just a quiet corner can go a long way toward creating positive momentum.

Each chapter will begin with the question "what went well?" Scan through your week -- or your recent memory -- and identify times when the particular weight or body issue you are dealing with was absent, or was not as strong. No problem exists 100% of the time. Ask yourself how you managed during these times. Take note of what inner and outer resources you used. On particularly bad weeks, consider how you were able to prevent things from getting worse. Your answers to these questions will reveal your unique areas of strength and competence.

By the time you have completed this book, you will have accomplished the following: created a Vision Statement, set one habit-change goal, one food-related goal, one activity goal, the Green for 15 challenge, and one goal of service to others. These goals will be small, manageable, and measurable. In addition, these small changes can produce big results! I hope you will find these exercises helpful as you begin the path of making peace with your weight. One step at a time.

1

Start from Where You Are

> IN THE BEGINNER'S MIND THERE ARE MANY POSSIBILITIES, BUT IN THE EXPERT'S THERE ARE FEW.
> SHUNRYU SUZUKI

How to Begin. Again.

When it comes to weight, our culture has it all backwards. Our bodies are the enemy. Our weight is to be feared. Food is a dangerous temptation. Exercise is a necessary evil. We beat our bodies into submission with workout routines we despise, or abuse ourselves through sedentary behavior. We label ourselves "bad" for indulging in rich desserts, and "good" for drinking green smoothies. We have lost touch with our internal signals of hunger and fullness. We have lost faith in our governing bodies, which come up with conflicting nutrition recommendations every few years. We mistrust the producers of our food, who seem to engineer food to create craving and dependence. We have become depleted and disillusioned with the lose it/gain it back again yo-yo of "diets." But worst of all: we no longer trust our bodies to guide us in the right direction.

How can we get back to a place of sanity? The ancient practice of mindfulness is the answer. Mindfulness will help you to tap into your own inner wisdom to 1) understand how maintaining a healthy weight is a "whole life issue" rather than a "diet and exercise" issue, and 2) reconnect with yourself so you can unlock the secret of permanent habit change.

The first step is to realize that all you will ever have is the present moment. As discouraged as you might feel--having tried many diets before--you can learn to cultivate what is known as "beginner's mind." The Zen Master Shunryu Suzuki is famous for saying: "In the beginner's mind there are many possibilities, in the expert's there are few."

Take a moment to contemplate this statement. It is quite the opposite of common wisdom, which holds that the expert is to be preferred over the novice. While experts certainly have a lot of knowledge and experience, they often lack possibility and energy. By allowing the truth of "beginner's mind" to permeate your consciousness, you can turn discouragement on its head. Beginner's mind is available to you every moment.

Life is full of setbacks--making peace with your weight is no different. It is a given that you will have setbacks, potholes, and bad days/weeks. What will set you up for success is how well you are able to access the energy of "beginner's mind." Rather than greeting each new beginning with a weary "not this again" sigh (and giving up!), you can see it as full of energy. We all have a limitless amount of beginnings, and each beginning always holds potent seeds of possibility.

Whether you are feeling bad about last night's binge or pessimistic about your twentieth time trying to lose weight, each new moment is a fresh place to start. It truly is the only moment we ever have. As you begin to practice mindfulness every day, you will train yourself to arrive in the present moment, each time afresh.

Mindful Life in Action: How I Found Zen

I am a lifelong spiritual seeker. Ever since I opened my first yoga book at the age of 14, I have gravitated to the life of the mind and the spirit. I have studied Christian mysticism, the yogic scriptures, the Tarot, Jungian psychology, western philosophy, shamanism, and Buddhism. However, it wasn't until I entered my first Zen temple that I became acquainted with the concept of beginner's mind. Zen was sparse, clean, and minimalist. There wasn't a book of scripture, prayer books, or music anywhere to be found. There were no decorations on the walls. There were simple dark brown cushions on the floor and a small vase of flowers--that was it. I wasn't greeted warmly by anyone, just silent smiles and bows. The instructions were to sit there, without moving, and count my breaths one through ten. When my mind drifted, start back at one. I don't think I ever got past two or three. It was my introduction to the present tense. One. One. One, two. One. One. When I experienced the present moment--over and over again--- I developed a visceral understanding of what it means to return to the eternal present, and of the expanse that can be found there. This cannot be taught. It must be experienced. In the stark and silent Zen temple, I embarked upon the somewhat tedious journey toward the present, aware that I would always be a beginner. And that was a good thing.

What is Mindfulness?

Mindfulness is the nonjudgmental awareness of the present moment and its thoughts, emotions, and needs. It is a skill that can be developed with regular practice. The first part of that definition—nonjudgmental ---entails creating an attitude of acceptance about circumstances, reactions, feelings, mental states, and relationships. As you continue to practice the skill of mindfulness, you develop a "witness consciousness" whereby you observe yourself. You observe your own mind---the content of your thoughts, emotions, and needs. You observe your own habits, taking note of habitual patterns, thoughts, and behaviors. You observe your own "self-talk," i.e., what you are telling yourself about your experience. Finally, you begin to observe the various areas of your life and how they fit together.

Mindful Life Weight Loss

Mindfulness is like a muscle. The more you use it, the stronger it becomes. Mindfulness is also like shining a light. The moment you shine the light of awareness onto something, it is the beginning of change. It is half the battle.

How Does Mindfulness Work?

Mindfulness helps us to better understand the complex nature of our behavior---what is really going on. Much of our behavior happens automatically, beneath the level of our consciousness and intentionality. When we become an observer of our own minds, we develop greater self-awareness of these automatic habits. Based on this self-knowledge, we are better prepared to meet challenges and make decisions that are more in line with our goals. We become actors, rather than reactors.

We Are Not Our Thoughts

Too often, our thoughts are judgmental and negative. We may be harsh with ourselves, proclaiming that we "should" be a certain weight, or "should" be able to resist unhealthy foods. We may be pessimistic, telling ourselves that this weight loss plan will fail just like all the others. We may "catastrophize," believing that one small mistake will result in utter failure. Mindfulness helps us to realize that we are not our thoughts, and to look upon the totality of our experiences with kindness. One participant reacted in horror when she turned the light of mindfulness onto her own self-talk. She observed, "If we were to talk to any other human being the way we talk to ourselves, it would be abuse."

Mindful Life Weight Loss

Thich Nhat Hanh uses the metaphor of a mother tending to a crying child. The calm, stable, and loving presence of the mother soothes the crying infant. This is how the energy of mindfulness works: it "holds" the moment with compassion and presence. In so doing, it transforms the moment. Next time you feel shameful or judgmental towards yourself for going on an eating binge, or for gaining weight, think of the mother and child metaphor. How might this change things?

Mindful Life in Action: How I Loosened the Identification with My Thoughts

Several years ago, my spiritual travels brought me to an ashram in upstate New York. I spent one summer attending weekly meditation instruction with a senior disciple of the guru who had founded the ashram. He was long deceased, and his disciples were continuing the lineage. The teacher was an older woman-- very humble-- who patiently instructed us to become a witness to our own thoughts: a silent and still observer. She had even made a recording to guide people through the process of witnessing our breath, bodily sensations, sounds in the environment, and thoughts. I have listened to this recording more times than I can count. She frequently told us "You are not your body or your mind." It was a profound shift for me to discover the spaciousness of the witnessing process. I don't have to believe every thought I have, nor do I have to act on them. I remember

Mindful Life Weight Loss

meditating in the ashram's meditation room on hot Saturday afternoons, feeling the freedom and lightness that comes with this realization. It has been years since I've been back there, but I've carried the witnessing practice into my daily life. It has given me the space to move from automatic reaction to conscious decision.

Starting a Mindfulness Practice

Starting a "mindfulness practice" is the only prerequisite to beginning the Mindful Life Weight Loss program. If that is new to you, it's not as daunting as it sounds. Although I followed the path of Zen temples and yoga ashrams, you don't have to. Mindfulness is a skill that can fit in with any world view or religion. It is pragmatic and adaptable.

Think of any skill you have ever tried to learn. Whether it was cooking, dancing, or driving a car, it was necessary to practice that skill regularly so you could see improvement. Mindfulness is no different. You will set aside a small amount of time daily to practice your new skill. Like anything else, you will be bad at it at first, but you will improve with practice. The good news is that it does not require a large investment of time to begin a mindfulness practice. Start with a mere three to five minutes a day.

This is mind training. Our minds are like puppies, always chasing after the next new thing--following every enticing thought, becoming wrapped up in fleeting emotions, and mired in worn out story lines. When you watch your "puppy mind" running in circles and chasing every object (even its own tail), you realize that you have a choice.

Three Mindfulness Practices to Get You Started

The Ten Breaths Practice. In this practice, maintain an awareness of the breath going in and out of your nostrils. Pay attention to the breath as if it is the most fascinating event you have ever witnessed, noting the temperature of the air, the feeling of it going in and out, the pace of your breathing, and any other detail. When your attention wanders from the breath---which it inevitably will---gently bring it back. The breath is your anchor to the present moment.

Journal Practice. This is a good practice for those who like to do something. Choose a notebook that you will use exclusively for this practice. Set a timer for three to five minutes and begin to write freely whatever is on your mind. Check in with your self-talk, emotional state, and goals. Writing is an excellent exercise in mindfulness. Many people also find keeping a food journal helps them to become mindful of their eating habits.

Labeling the Moment Practice. In this practice, taught by Thich Nhat Hanh, you mentally tell yourself what you are doing as a way of arriving more fully into the present moment. An example of this is: "I am walking, and I know that I am walking." You can also do this with your breathing. This is my personal favorite. I say, "Breathing in, I know I am breathing in. Breathing out, I know I am breathing out" with each in-breath and out-breath. Continue this exercise for three to five minutes.

Mindful Life Weight Loss

You can use any or all of these as a way of bringing nonjudgmental awareness into your daily life. However, the best way to learn mindfulness techniques is to practice with a teacher. Check out local meditation or yoga classes, many of which are free or low cost. Learning from a teacher helps to address any questions that may arise as you get started.

You can also search on YouTube for mindfulness instruction, or download free mindfulness apps. Many reputable teachers, such as Thich Nhat Hanh, Jon Kabat Zinn, and Jack Kornfield, have free instructional videos and guided mindfulness exercises. It is very helpful to begin a mindfulness practice by having the voice of a teacher guide you through the process, rather than simply reading instructions.

During the few minutes of mindfulness practice, you will become more and more skilled at sitting still and not reacting to the whims of thought, sensation, and emotion. When a powerful emotion comes over you, you simply watch it rise, crest, and fall like a wave in the ocean. When an uncomfortable physical sensation arises---like an itch--you sit through it and realize that it is not an emergency. You begin to tolerate discomfort and distress, and this becomes a valuable skill when trying to change habits. You train your unruly puppy into a valuable service dog, able to change habits and achieve goals. When you cultivate the skill of mindful awareness, your mind becomes your greatest ally in your weight loss efforts.

Mindful Life Weight Loss

Mindful Life in Action: How I Learned to Become Comfortable in Uncomfortable Situations

Learning to tolerate distress has been one of the most valuable lessons I have learned. I was introduced to the concept of becoming comfortable in uncomfortable situations when I started training in martial arts. At the age of 38, I grew tired of the gym and signed up for an Aikido class. Aikido is a martial art that focuses on throwing people, similar to Judo. Simply walking into the dojo was uncomfortable, as I was the only female, and an older one at that. Having to practice techniques in close contact with others, learning to do things I had never done before---such as being thrown to the ground---and having somewhat painful techniques performed on me, was extremely uncomfortable. Yet, each day I showed up, in spite of the stomach butterflies, because I understood that this "distress tolerance" was somehow an important skill. Also, paradoxically, Aikido was a great deal of fun. Aikido taught me that I did not have to react to every negative thing that occurred in my physical and mental environment. I learned patience, and in that patience, I could make choices. Choices more aligned with my goals and values. This has been especially important in helping me to deal with emotional eating. Rather than reach for food to soothe painful feelings, I can tolerate them and ride them out like a wave. Aikido, yoga, and all martial arts are considered "moving meditation" and are

Mindful Life Weight Loss

excellent ways of training our bodies and minds to not be so reactive to the distresses of life.

Take a moment now to commit to three to five minutes a day to practice the skill of mindfulness. Think of the best time in your schedule---whether it is the morning before you get out of bed, in the evening when you are unwinding, or some other point in the day. Whatever you choose, try to make it a consistent time every day. Treat this time with the same respect you would have for an important appointment. It is the single greatest investment you can have in your own health.

Setting a "Sacred Space"

After choosing a daily time for your mindfulness practice, you should set aside a designated space. At the very least, your space should be quiet and allow you to sit comfortably with a straight back. Some people like to order special meditation cushions, but all you really need is a chair. During my time as a commuter, I was able to maintain a mindfulness practice on the train by using my iPod and a downloaded meditation audio file. I also maintained a mindfulness practice in my parked car during another busy period of my life. With some creativity, you can maintain your practice in even less than optimal circumstances.

Even if your space doubles as something else (your desk, kitchen table, a commuter train, etc.) make the space in some way "special" for your mindfulness practice. Carrying a special stone, wearing a particular piece of jewelry, or beginning your practice with some relaxing music are ways to differentiate your space if you are not at home. If you are at home, perhaps place an object there, that has significance to you such as a memento, seashell, picture, or rosary/meditation beads. A beautiful object from nature, such as flowers or a plant, can help in creating a positive mood. Some people like to create an altar with meaningful objects, or burn incense. If this helps you, that would be great. However, it is not necessary in the beginning. The idea is to find a simple and easy way to create the feeling that your mindfulness practice is something important and in some way sacred.

Performing your practice in the same place every day will help to accumulate momentum and energy. Think of the feeling when you enter a church, temple, or meditation center. The place has absorbed the energy of so many people that it resonates. It makes it easier to become quiet inside. The designated space will cue you into your practice and make it easier for you to continue. Some people even find that they look forward to their little space each day as a refuge from the busyness and stresses of life.

During our Mindful Life groups, we begin each session with a meditation bell and three minutes of silence. Many people find it helpful to cue their mindfulness practice with the sound of a meditation bell. You can download meditation bells and timers for your phone or find them on YouTube. Use the beautiful, reverberating sound of the bell to cue

Mindful Life Weight Loss

yourself that it is time to settle in and begin your practice.

Action Steps:

Mindfulness Exercise:

Take a moment and experiment with compassionate awareness. Set a timer, close your eyes, and spend 3 minutes watching your own thoughts, bodily sensations, and emotions. Don't try to change anything. Just observe. This will be how you begin each subsequent chapter.

Some guiding questions are:

What thoughts pass through my mind?

What am I feeling right now?

How does my body feel?

What is my breathing like? Shallow? Deep?

What sounds do I hear in the room at this moment? What do I smell?

Are there any recurring messages I tell myself ("self-talk")?

Take note of whether you were kind to yourself, or whether you were self-critical. Record any other observations here:

2

What is a Mindful Life?

> **MINDFULNESS IS ABOUT LOVE AND LOVING LIFE. WHEN YOU CULTIVATE THIS LOVE, IT GIVES YOU CLARITY AND COMPASSION FOR LIFE, AND YOUR ACTIONS HAPPEN IN ACCORDANCE WITH THAT.**
> **JON KABAT ZINN**

Begin practicing three minutes of silence.

How was your week?

What went well for you this week? How did you accomplish that?

Mindful living is a new way of being. You have probably been on many diets, and found that they work while you are on them, but then the weight comes back when old habits return. Diets don't work because they don't address the fundamental lifestyle change that creates new, healthy habits. A new way of being is the only way to end your war with weight, and live a healthier and happier life.

Diets, and most conventional weight loss programs, put you at war with your appetite and your habits. They operate from a place of "don't" rather than a place of "do." A place of "what's wrong" rather than "what's right." After a certain period of time, it becomes impossible to sustain the effort required to overcome food cravings, count calories, and maintain rigorous food diaries. Depleted and discouraged, people abandon their diets and gain the weight right back.

This war requires the finite reserve of willpower, which only weakens each time you use it. Think of willpower as a bucket of water. Each time you dip into it, it gets lower and lower. When you try to lose weight primarily through avoiding certain foods and behaviors, you drain your supply of willpower. There is a better way to effectively understand and unwind problematic habits in a way that does not require deprivation and willpower.

Mindful Life in Action: Joe's Small Changes and Big Results

Joe's participation in the Mindful Life program required very little of what would traditionally be called willpower. He had gained and lost the same 50 pounds

Mindful Life Weight Loss

many times in his life. This time, he was doing something different. Joe made extremely small changes in several areas of his life (mindfulness, diet, exercise, relationships, and outdoor time). He would lose a pound a week, and then plateau for several weeks. Then he would lose again in the same gradual manner. We worked with Joe to understand that plateaus are fine as long as you are committed to the process. Thus, Joe never felt pressured to make changes faster than was realistic. He never saw the plateau as a reason to give up. He remarked that this was the easiest weight loss program he had ever followed. The long-term process allowed Joe to solidify his new habits so there was no danger of going back to his old lifestyle.

This program operates from a systems theory perspective that sees the whole person in the context of their whole lives. Systems theory, discussed in greater detail in Chapters 8 and 9, is a way of looking at the world that sees everything as a relationship among parts. Weight cannot be addressed solely from one perspective. It must be addressed in proper context. We don't target isolated habits, and attempt to change them. Instead, we take a wide angle view, consider the precise inter-relationship of different parts of our lives , and strategically target small habits in key areas. By the end of this book, you will have gained momentum with five small habit change goals. And, like Joe, your transformation can be effortless and gradual.

Mindful Life Weight Loss

What is a "Mindful Life?"

A Mindful Life balances the precise inter-relationships between the Five Areas of Weight Loss. They are:

1. The basic practice of mindfulness: nonjudgmental awareness of the present moment and its thoughts, emotions, and needs. Basic mindfulness entails taking a pause and tuning into the present moment, and the thoughts, emotions, and needs that arise. It is an increase in awareness and clarity. This book will help you to develop a greater awareness of your internal and external environment and the resulting habits that have contributed to weight gain. You will learn how the brain works to form habits, and the science behind changing habits.
2. A healthy diet. There is no need to go on a specific "diet." Rather, you should choose a healthy, balanced diet that avoids deprivation, quick weight loss, drugs, or fads. The diet you choose should be something that you feel is sustainable over time, even after you have lost the weight. A healthy diet consists primarily of unprocessed, whole foods, i.e., those foods found on the perimeter of your supermarket. Switching to simply prepared unprocessed foods can help your body to regulate hunger and satiety naturally.
3. Increased activity and movement. A Mindful Life does not require extreme exercise, but over time, you will become less sedentary and more active. You will explore exercise that is organic and incremental to your life, and --

most importantly-- that you enjoy. If you find that you simply don't like to work out, this book will help you to add natural activity to your daily life in a way that works for you.
4. Relational thinking. Systems theory is seeing the whole picture rather than just the parts. Each part of your life relates to other parts, and they all impact your weight loss. Systems theory can explain yo-yo dieting and how to address it. In this book, you will understand the big picture of weight gain and weight loss. Plus, it's vital to explore how interpersonal relationships can help you to become accountable and why it might seem that others are sabotaging your weight loss. As a result, you can choose how and when to include family and friends in your weight loss goals.
5. Nature. We spend more time indoors than ever before. Many of us, especially children, spend our days moving from building to car to building. The glow of our screens has replaced the light of day. This book explores our culture's increased screen time and the disappearance of work/life balance. You will become more aware of your habits surrounding screen time and make incremental changes— and learn how spending as little as 15 minutes a day outdoors can help you to decrease stress and improve well-being.

Letting Go of the Story Line

One of the first things you will notice as you embark upon a Mindful Life is that much of your mental chatter is comprised of recurring narratives you tell yourself. These are your familiar stories. You may see yourself as a persistent victim of circumstance, or as a survivor and warrior, or any number of "roles." The raw data of your life is given a specific meaning, and that meaning tends to take on a life of its own. It may even become your identity. These stories become problematic when they are fossilized into an identity from which you cannot break free. Here are a few examples. Do any of them sound familiar?

I am a victim.
I have no willpower.
The world is against me.
I am alone.
Nothing ever works out for me.
I start out strong but always lose steam.
I am a fat person.
I cannot control myself around food.
I am not athletic.
I am not the type of person who exercises.
I cannot lose weight.
I always gain the weight back.

What is your recurring storyline? Take a few moments to contemplate this question. Think of your struggles with weight, and what kind of narrative you have been telling yourself.

Adopting a mindfulness practice will help you to recognize these familiar story lines, and most importantly, help you to realize they are not reality. They are merely story lines, and story lines can be rewritten.

Mindful Life Weight Loss

Mindful Life in Action: Robert the "Couch Potato" turned Yogi

Robert was a self-described "couch potato" in his early forties who had spent most of his life as a sedentary person. He was an avid video game player, and movie aficionado. Robert was very passionate about his hobbies, but they were all sedentary. Robert's sedentary life, combined with a diet high in processed food and animal products, left Robert with a weight problem as well as diabetes. As part of his weight loss plan, Robert took up yoga. Through his months of dedicated yoga practice---sometimes seven days a week---Robert brought his weight into a healthy range and reversed his diabetes. Robert also transformed his life narrative. He now took up the identity of "yogi" and fully embraced the yoga lifestyle, still maintaining his hobbies but not as center stage. His daily life choices were dictated by this new identity. Not only did Robert change his eating and exercise regimen, but he also dramatically reduced his alcohol consumption. His new life narrative of health-loving yogi was more joyful and vibrant than his former narrative. It was quite a transformation.

Seeing Solutions

The Mindful Life Weight Loss program is a solution-focused approach. In the early 1980s, psychotherapists Steve De Shazer and Insoo Kim Berg created an innovative form of brief psychotherapy called Solution-Focused Brief Therapy. De Shazer became famous for saying: "Problem talk creates problems. Solution talk creates solutions." During their sessions with clients, they did not ask about the past, or open old wounds. They believed that it was not necessary to know anything about the origin of the problem in order to arrive at a solution. They were mavericks in their belief that the problem and the solution were not necessarily related.

They helped clients to see their current life with new eyes. With this "solution focus," people were guided to direct their attention to times when their problems were not occurring. As bad as our problems may be, no problem occurs 100% of the time. There are always exceptions, and problem-free times. This approach asks: what is different about those times, and how can that be amplified?

De Shazer and Berg shifted the focus to these problem-free exceptions, and inquired with genuine curiosity how the client managed to have those exceptions. The talk during the therapy hour (and for them it was often much shorter than an hour) focused entirely on times when the problem was not occurring. It was a revolutionary, uplifting way of solving problems.

They sought to build up the solutions rather than "solve the problems" by helping people to envision their lives without their problems, and take small steps in that direction. This model of psychotherapy has also influenced the coaching world, and has proven very helpful in the Mindful Life Weight Loss program. Focusing on what went well, exceptions to the problem, times when you managed to prevent something from getting even worse, and signs that you are moving closer to your preferred future are all hallmarks of the Mindful Life approach.

Mindful Life in Action: Jessica's Solutions

Jessica was a night-time binge eater. She ate as a way of coping with painful emotions. She would restrict her food intake all day so that she could binge at night, after coming home from work. She was currently in psychotherapy to deal with this issue, but was making little progress. She had also visited several nutritionists who simply reiterated what she already knew: starving herself all day only triggered night-time binge eating. Jessica knew that she needed to eat regular meals, but could not take this very big step. When I began working with her, I gently drew her attention to moments when she was either not starving herself during the day, or times at night when she was able to stop her binges earlier than usual, or to consume slightly less food. In the beginning, I worked with Jessica several times per week. I asked her "what went well?" and she was often at a loss to respond. She would report what a "bad night" she had, or how much she ate. Buried in the report of what when wrong would be a glimmer of hope: she threw out a box of cookies after eating half of them, or she woke up and had a small breakfast. I would "freeze frame" those moments and ask her how she managed to do that. What inner resources did she use to be able to stop herself from eating a whole box of cookies? Jessica shared that she relied upon her faith in God, and upon a healthy dose of fear that binges were harming her health. This moved Jessica out of a mindset of "I cannot control my binge eating" to one of "I can control myself." Slowly, Jessica's successes increased. She amplified her faith in God, began praying more, and became more involved with her community of faith, thus giving her many opportunities for the connection she craved. She began eating three meals a day. Not once did we ever delve into her past, or seek to unearth painful emotions. We focused on solutions, not problems.

Every problem contains the seeds of the solution. The trick is in training your mind to focus on the solution, and to build out the skills and resiliencies that are already present in your life and environment, as Jessica did.

Think of a time when you had an eating binge, or went off your healthy eating plan. Surely, buried within that time, you will find a moment where things could have gotten worse--but did not-- or where you were able to stop yourself (perhaps you only ate half of the cake). These moments may not look like successes to you, but inspect them closely. How were you able to do what you did? How can you move one step closer to having more of those moments?

The Vision Statement: Your Contract with Yourself.

Mindful Life Weight Loss

A clear, tangible statement of your weight loss vision is an essential first step of a Mindful Life. It tells you, in great detail, where you are going, why you want to go there, and how you will get there. Think of it as the map, or GPS, of your journey. A good Vision Statement has three main components: Past, Present, and Future. Write your answers to these sections in the Vision Statement at the end of the chapter.

Past: Take a moment to consider why you picked up this book. Why do you want to lose weight? Consider what has brought you to the point where you are ready to make changes in your life. Is it health-related? Job-related? Has your family motivated you? Are you unhappy with the way you have been feeling? Whatever it is, include it in your statement.

Present: A good Vision Statement will take into account how you want to feel now. Not today, tomorrow, or next year. Right now. Aim for the feeling you want to have as a person living a healthy life. Often, these are exactly the feelings that you are trying to access with food. They may be: relaxed, satisfied, energetic, excited, in control, safe, loved, peaceful, etc. You need not wait until you are at your desired weight to feel the way you want to feel. You will develop new habits that give you access to these feelings right now, but in a healthy way.

Future. This is the nuts and bolts of how you will achieve weight loss. This is for small, measurable, attainable goals in the areas of habits, and you will add to it as you add small goals along the way. This could be an amount of weight to lose, as long as it is measured out in small, achievable increments (i.e. "I will lose one pound this week."). It could also be any of the habit changes that we work on throughout this program. You will add new goals to the third section each week, so leave these blank for now.

This Vision Statement will remain with you through this journey. Write it down, print it out, make copies, and put it in as many places as possible. It is an evolving document that you will add to over the course of this book.

If you are tempted to skip this part, don't. Just as you wouldn't enter into a business arrangement without a contract, don't begin this important process without formalizing it in writing.

Tell as many people as possible. The more you see it and speak it, the more real it becomes. What we focus on gains both power and momentum. The more you integrate your Vision Statement into your daily consciousness, the more powerful it will become.

During times when your motivation falters, look at your Vision Statement to re-charge and re-focus.

Your Shadow Vision: The Reasons You Don't Want to Lose Weight

Of equal importance to your Vision Statement is your "Shadow Vision." The concept of the shadow is associated with Carl Jung, but also appears in many wisdom traditions. We all have parts of ourselves that

Mindful Life Weight Loss

are disowned, repressed, and hidden. Everything that is light has its corresponding shadow. We embrace the light--the healthy goals, motivation, and positive affirmations. We repress the darkness--the ambivalence, resistance, and ulterior motives.

Mindfulness allows us to examine those shadows, learn from them, and integrate them into the wholeness of our experience. When it comes to losing weight, if we don't address the underlying reasons why we don't want to lose weight, those reasons will sabotage our efforts later on.

People have expressed various shadow reasons in our program. For some, excess weight is a protective and insulating mechanism. For others, excess weight provides an excuse for not moving forward in some area of life: "I'll look for a new job as soon as I lose weight...". For couples, weight might symbolize a barrier to intimacy, or be used to test a partner's unconditional love. These shadow reasons are unique to each person. Mindful awareness can help you uncover yours, and integrate them into your overall plan. Simply bringing these reasons into compassionate awareness activates this integration.

Take a moment to reflect on why you do not want to lose weight. Know that it is normal to have mixed feelings, and be kind to yourself. Some helpful prompts are:

I don't want to lose weight because....

Staying at this weight allows me to.....

Mindful Life Weight Loss

Action Steps:

Post your evolving Vision Statement in as many places as you can.

This week, simply observe your habits surrounding food. Some questions to consider are:

When am I most likely to overeat (evening, late afternoons, weekends, etc)?

What foods do I typically binge on? Are there any similarities to these foods
i.e. high sugar, carbohydrate, fast foods, etc.)

What situations are likely to cause overeating?

Are there any people in my life that I am more likely to overeat with than others?

Do I tend to eat alone?

When in my life did my eating begin to become a source of struggle?

Was it in response to a major life event (job, divorce, childbirth, death)?

What feelings tend to trigger overeating?

What is the reward--or payoff--of my habitual behaviors?

Mindful Life Weight Loss

You can write any other observations here:

There are no right or wrong answers. See what you discover.

Don't try to change anything. Simply observe and take note. We will examine how to change habits in the next chapter.

VISION STATEMENT

I want to lose weight because:

1.

2.

3.

I want to feel:

1.

2.

3.

I will: (these goals will be filled in as you progress through the book):

1. Initial habit change goal (or could be pounds you want to lose):

2. Food goal:

3. Activity goal:

4. Green for 15:

5. One goal that benefits others:

3

Setting Goals

> IN ASIAN LANGUAGES, THE WORD FOR 'MIND' AND THE WORD FOR 'HEART' ARE SAME. SO IF YOU'RE NOT HEARING MINDFULNESS IN SOME DEEP WAY AS HEARTFULNESS, YOU'RE NOT REALLY UNDERSTANDING IT. COMPASSION AND KINDNESS TOWARDS ONESELF ARE INTRINSICALLY WOVEN INTO IT. YOU COULD THINK OF MINDFULNESS AS WISE AND AFFECTIONATE ATTENTION.
> JON KABAT ZINN

Begin by practicing three minutes of silence.

How was your week?

What went well for you this week (i.e., times when the problem was not occurring)? How did you accomplish that?

What was your experience with posting your Vision Statement around your household?

How did your family/spouse/friends react?

What food habits did you notice as you did the homework?

Habits

Aristotle has said, "We are what we repeatedly do." Much of our everyday behavior happens beneath the level of our intention. It happens by habit. Evolution has wired us to act this way-- automatically, out of habit. This is a particularly efficient way of surviving. If we had to "re-invent the wheel" each time we performed an action, life would be extremely cumbersome and impractical. Our ancestors would not have been able to be efficient builders, for example, if they had to intentionally perform every action while constructing shelter from the elements. Habit allowed them to efficiently and quickly perform the necessary tasks for survival. Automatic behavior has its place. However, our automatic habits are harming our health.

Habits have a very simple structure. There is the trigger, the habitual action itself, and the reward. Mindfulness interrupts the habit cycle at each point. It helps you to examine your triggers and their context. It helps you to consciously examine and evaluate the action itself. And finally, it helps you to assess the reward--or payoff--and find alternative ways of meeting this need. The only antidote to mindless automatic behavior is mindfulness.

Mindful Life Weight Loss

Habits are like a path through the woods. The more the path is walked on, the easier it becomes to continue to walk on it. The more we perform a certain habit, the more likely we are to do that habit again and again. This is what happens in our brain "circuitry" with repeated behaviors.

The good news is that our brain is not a fixed, solid organ. Our brains are plastic and flexible. They can change---and "rewire"---in response to usage and experience. This is called neuroplasticity, and it occurs through the entire human lifespan. You can teach an old dog new tricks. Jane was able to reverse a lifetime of social eating through the process of mindfully identifying her triggers and formulating a realistic alternative plan.

Mindful Life in Action: Jane's Social Eating

Jane was a 60-year-old engineer who struggled with social eating. When she was alone in her home, she had a healthy routine that was both comfortable and sustainable. However, when Jane found herself in a social situation, she would eat far beyond her comfort level. This would happen at work functions, dinner parties, family gatherings, and holidays. Using the skill of mindfulness, Jane was able to tune into how she was feeling during social situations and identify that she felt anxious and uneasy. She was able to target the trigger in the habit cycle: social situations. Social anxiety triggered eating, which served the purpose of soothing the anxiety and making the social situations more bearable for her. However, Jane later regretted her eating behavior, which would often

Mindful Life Weight Loss

include lots of high-sugar desserts. During the holiday season, Jane would often gain weight. Through enacting the Mindful Life program, Jane made it through a very busy holiday season with a stable weight. Once she identified the trigger, she was able to formulate a strategy to interrupt the habit cycle. She decided to "have a plan" for every social occasion. She would make sure she was not too hungry before. She would always have a glass of mineral water with lemon in her hand to sip on, and she stuck to a "one plate" rule. Jane also did a visualization before each event, where she would completely relax and visualize herself enacting her plan and being successful. However, without mindfulness, Jane would not have been able to interrupt the habit cycle and create this new habit.

Take a moment and list one habit in your current lifestyle that is not helpful to you on your path toward weight loss. This can be a habit that you observed since beginning this book or anything that comes to mind. Think of habits surrounding food, movement, work, relationships, or any other area of your lifestyle. Remember, weight loss is not just about food or exercise. It is a lifestyle issue. Therefore, an unhelpful habit in one area (overwork, conflictual relationships, etc.) could indirectly lead to weight gain. List your habit here:

Like Jane, in shining the light of mindful awareness on this habit, you have taken the first step on the path of change. Far from being a passive act, this is a powerful activating force toward achieving your goal. Each subsequent step will help to "rewire" your brain

Mindful Life Weight Loss

to form a new habit. These new habits will lead you on a path toward greater happiness and health.

This will be uncomfortable at first. It is important to recognize this fact. Many people are initially very excited about changing a habit only to experience the discomfort of trying to maintain the new behavior. This is normal. It is simply your brain doing what your brain does.

Likewise, your life has functioned in much the same way for quite some time. There is a natural resistance to change, called homeostasis, which we will discuss in detail in Chapter 8.

But for now, remember, the path of least resistance is the path that has been worn smooth with travel. That path has led you to this book. Now, you are forging a new path through untrodden terrain. When you feel the initial discomfort about changing a habit, tell yourself that it is normal and will become easier over time.

Common wisdom says that it takes between 30 and 45 days to solidify a new habit. Sometimes it takes longer if people take a few steps back every now and again (this is totally normal, and does not mean you should give up). It is vitally important to maintain a support system of like-minded people during this time. It will also help to post your Vision Statement in as many places as possible.

The best way to change a habit is by taking small steps. Sudden, drastic changes to your lifestyle will create a strong push-back. You should not try to overhaul every area of your life, or embark upon sweeping, drastic changes. Small steps, however, rarely stay small. They have a tendency to create their own positive momentum and lead to bigger steps, and eventually the achievement of your ultimate goal.

Mindful Life in Action: Small Steps to a Big Goal

Jeff was a 50-year-old stay at home dad who was a self-described "sugar addict." He referred to sugary drinks and foods as his "drug of choice" that gave him energy to get through the day. Jeff made it clear that he was not going to give up sugar---ever---but he nevertheless wanted to lose weight and regain some control over his eating. We worked with Jeff to set and achieve small, manageable goals, such as replacing only one sugary snack per day with fresh fruit. However, after only two months Jeff had incrementally expanded his goals with each new success, and had even replaced his soda habit with sparkling water and a splash of fruit juice. When I asked Jeff if he would ever have imagined coming as far as he had, he replied that he would have thought it impossible. He took small steps and climbed a rather steep hill without even realizing it.

Setting and Achieving Goals

These small steps on the path of change take the form of goals. Many of us have mixed experiences with goals. Perhaps you have set a goal of "going to the gym" and watched it quickly lose steam. Perhaps you have had one too many New Year's resolutions fail before Valentine's Day. But you can stop this cycle of frustration by keeping a process-focused mindset and understanding the dynamics of goal setting.

There is a simple science to goal achievement: think small, measurable, attainable, and accountable.

Goals should be small, not big. They should be challenging enough to be worth pursuing, but small enough to be plausible. Rather than saying "This year I will go to the gym three times a week," it is better to say "This week I will go for a 15 minute walk after lunch for three days." With the latter goal, not only are you choosing a less ambitious goal, but you are choosing a more attainable goal. If you are not already in the habit of working out, vowing to go to the gym three times a week for the rest of the year is unrealistic. Not impossible, but unlikely. Changing the goal from "going to the gym" to "walking" moves the goal closer to what you are already likely to perform. If you are more likely to carry out the goal, you will succeed. Then you will create positive momentum and build confidence. You will also build a new habit that will someday be just as natural and effortless as your current unhelpful habits.

Success breeds success. Once you have achieved some of your smaller goals, you will begin to feel like you have unlocked the secret to goal achievement and then will want to move onto bigger goals. As one of our participants declared, "I feel like I can accomplish anything with this process!"

Additionally, linking the new goal to an action that is already part of your routine makes it more likely to achieve the goal. Going to lunch will be the trigger for the new behavior (taking a walk). Even better would be to link the new behavior to an already existing behavior that you enjoy. Perhaps you enjoy shopping. You can then add "going for a walk" to each trip to the mall.

Make sure your goal is measurable: quantify it. Say how many minutes you will walk, how many pounds you want to lose this week, by how much you will reduce your sugar intake, by how much you will reduce eating out, etc.

You may wonder if such small goals are likely to have a real effect. Perhaps you have one hundred pounds to lose. Can adding a few walks every week really help? The answer is unequivocally "yes." Systems theory states that a small change in one part of the system can produce results in other areas. The reason is it does not stop there. Every drop has a ripple effect outward to other areas of your life.

Let's look at the many ways that adding a small goal like a 15 minute walk can have a ripple effect on your entire lifestyle. In making that one change, you are already increasing your level of activity. You may notice a slightly lower number on the scale, improved muscle tone, and an increase in energy. Spending time outdoors will be both energizing and relaxing, and have the added bonus of reducing sedentary screen time and stress. Stress-related eating might decrease as a result. Who knows, you may take that walk with a co-worker or family member, thus adding a satisfying relational component and increasing accountability (you wouldn't want to let your co-worker down by canceling the walk). You might also begin to make changes in your diet, realizing that you no longer want to eat as much because you don't want to disrupt your positive momentum. Finally, if you are practicing mindfulness, that 15-minute walk can truly be a fulfilling experience.

Consider the habit you listed earlier that led to your weight gain. Now, think of a goal that can be linked to that habit.

Decide if that goal is small and attainable enough to be realistic. You may not be able to undo the entire habit yet, but can target one small part of it. Some helpful questions are:

How much of a deviation from my usual routine is this goal?

Is this goal linked to anything I already do or enjoy?

If it is a "pounds lost" goal, is it healthy and realistic?

How can I measure this goal (having a number is helpful)?

Is the time frame for this goal brief enough (a good rule is to set the goal for no longer than one week's time, and then refreshing the goal each week)?

Mindful Life in Action: How Sarah Set a Small Goal

Mindful Life Weight Loss

Sarah was a 25-year-old college student who was in the habit of drinking sugary soft drinks throughout the day. In addition, she snacked on candy, chips, and cookies. Sarah wanted to limit her consumption of sugar in order to lose weight. Rather than deciding to eliminate soda, candy, chips, and cookies from her diet at once, Sarah came up with the following goal: "I will replace one sugary drink with a glass of water each day this week." The next week, after she had achieved this goal (which she found easily attainable), Sarah felt ready to replace all of her soft drinks with sparkling water and lemon. Sarah was participating in an online weight loss group where members were encouraged to post pictures engaging in their healthy habits. Sarah became excited to post selfies of her drinking mineral water spritzers, or water mixed with lemons and other fruit. Sarah's friends were also inspired to drink water instead of soft drinks when they dined out with her.

Now it is time to write down your small, measurable, and attainable goal. Remember, change takes time. Rather than trying to change the entire behavior (which was years in the making), address a small part of it. Rather than eliminating all sugar and junk food from her diet, Sarah started by eliminating soft drinks.

My goal:

Mindful Life Weight Loss

Revisit your goal to make sure it is small, measurable, and attainable. A rule of thumb is that it is better to attempt to do less, rather than to overextend yourself. This way, you will be guaranteed success and positive momentum, rather than the opposite.

Write this goal on your Vision Statement.

The final factor that will aid in goal achievement is accountability. Post your goal in as many places as possible (post-it notes, reminders on your phone, sharing on social media, etc.). Share the goal with the group (or a friend/family member) as well. Feel free to enlist a friend's help. Perhaps you can say "I'm really trying to stop drinking soda with lunch. If you see me grabbing a Coke, could you remind me to drink water?"

Deepak Chopra has said "Success comes when people act together. Failure tends to happen alone." When I embarked upon daily walking, my daughter helped to keep me accountable.

Sarah was able to receive support from her online friends who were all trying to lose weight.

Remember:

Set reminders on your phone
Write it on a post-it note and put it everywhere
Enlist the support of this group
Team up with a coach or trainer
Ask for help from your friends and family
Use social media

Mindful Life Weight Loss

Think of some other creative ways you can enhance accountability. List them here:

Environmental Modification

Modifying your surroundings is a way to create an environment that is consciously conducive to success. If a goal is to decrease consumption of a certain food, for example, you can take steps to rid your home environment of that food. If your goal is to avoid eating at restaurants for one week, you can spend some time pre-cooking or pre-packing meals for the week so you always have food ready.

Motivation, by nature, fluctuates in response to any number of factors. Tiredness, stress, the weather...all of these can impact your ability to succeed at your goal. Take advantage of times when your motivation is strong to set your environment up for success. That way, your success is less dependent of the ebbs and flows of motivation.

Brainstorm ways that you can modify your environment to increase your success. Write your ideas here:

Mindful Life Weight Loss

Mindful Life in Action: Mark's Locking the Pantry

Mark was a 55-year-old science teacher who labeled himself a "night time grazer." His eating habits were great during the day, but at night, he felt a complete loss of control that had resulted in a significant weight gain over the years. He lived with his wife, who liked to keep the pantry stocked with snack foods. For Mark, access to an array of tempting foods was a trigger for him. He was not yet at a point where he felt he could be around snack foods without eating more than he wanted to. He and his wife came up with a plan to put all of the snack foods in one cabinet of the pantry. His wife would lock this cabinet after dinner. For Mark, this was enough to quell his trigger and allow his mind to focus on other things. While he wanted to reach a point where he did not need to modify the environment, this was an important first step to interrupt the habit cycle and begin to lose weight. Modifying the environment helped Mark to take the decision out of his hands when he felt his motivation was low or shaky.

How to Handle Setbacks and Fluctuating Motivation

Setbacks and fluctuating motivation are normal parts of the process of change. If they didn't happen, you wouldn't be changing. No one has ever achieved any goal without these two elements. Factor them in from the outset. That way, when they rear their little heads, you can smile and say "Hello, setback. Hello faltering motivation. I've been waiting for you." The real danger is that people interpret setbacks and fluctuating motivation as "failures." Then, they give up. They mistakenly assume they "lack willpower" or that something is wrong with them.

Instead, think back to what you have learned about mindfulness. Your focus should be on compassionate awareness, and being present with the totality of your experience. Welcome these visitors in with that same compassionate awareness. Be curious about what they have to teach you. Perhaps your latest setback contains a new insight into your behavior. Perhaps the ebb and flow of your motivation is your body's way of telling you to ease up on yourself, or slow down the process of change. Perhaps what you interpret as an ebb in motivation is really just another area of your life in need of attention. You might need to re-direct your attention temporarily to a work crisis or family emergency. Rest assured that if you become quiet inside, your innate inner wisdom will show you the way.

When you are able to integrate these phenomena compassionately into your experience as a whole, you are far more likely to continue onward with positive momentum. This is the nature of a process-focused approach, as opposed to simply focusing on goals.

This is one benefit of being part of a supportive community. When you are able to check in with others, they can provide important feedback and

Mindful Life Weight Loss

insight that you might not be considering. You will also be able to do the same for them.

Change Your Focus: Process vs. Goal

The "awareness" part of mindfulness is an evolving goal. We never arrive. The process is the destination. It will be your practice. Mindfulness is something you do-- over and over again.

Many people become very focused on their goal: to achieve a certain "ideal" weight or level of fitness. They direct all of their energy and effort toward this singular goal. Each pound lost is a step in the right direction. Each "bad week" where they gain weight is a disappointment and step backwards. Think of the cringe-worthy public weigh-ins in popular weight loss programs and TV reality shows. It may surprise you to learn that this goal-directed behavior is a surefire way to fail. It is not that goals in and of themselves are not useful, but rather that the bulk of your attention needs to be on your commitment to the process, not the specific goal.

Rather than focus on your ideal weight, direct your focus to the process of your mindfulness practice. This way you are not at the mercy of every up and down, but fully grounded and committed to the process of mindful living. You are better able to stay centered and grounded in the present moment--the only moment we have. It also allows you to handle setbacks and failures. How you handle setbacks and failures (which are inevitable) is one of the biggest indicators of whether you will ultimately be able to change your life for the better.

Mindful Life Weight Loss

Instead of seeing the inevitable ups and downs as obstacles to your goal and things to become discouraged about, your focus becomes the process of unfolding self-awareness. Each setback is an opportunity to gain insight and to improve your situation. Each moment becomes a fresh moment to practice compassionate awareness, rather than merely a rung on the ladder to your goal. Each failure contains within it seeds of the solution.

ACTION STEPS:

THIS WEEK YOU WILL ACHIEVE YOUR GOAL. AS AN EXERCISE IN MINDFULNESS, REWRITE YOUR GOAL HERE:

MY GOAL:

LIST THE WAY (OR WAYS) THAT YOU WILL BE ACCOUNTABLE FOR THIS GOAL:

LIST HOW YOU WILL CREATE AN ENVIRONMENT FOR SUCCESS:

AND DON'T FORGET TO ADD THIS GOAL TO YOUR VISION STATEMENT. REMEMBER TO KEEP YOUR VISION STATEMENT POSTED IN PROMINENT PLACES.

Mindful Life Weight Loss

AND GO....YOUR ACTION STEP IS TO ACHIEVE YOUR GOAL THIS WEEK. YOU CAN DO IT! ONE STEP AT A TIME.

4

Mindfulness and Food

> PEOPLE NEED TO KNOW THAT THEY HAVE ALL THE TOOLS WITHIN THEMSELVES. SELF-AWARENESS, WHICH MEANS AWARENESS OF THEIR BODY, AWARENESS OF THEIR MENTAL SPACE, AWARENESS OF THEIR RELATIONSHIPS - NOT ONLY WITH EACH OTHER, BUT WITH LIFE AND THE ECOSYSTEM.
> DEEPAK CHOPRA

Begin with three minutes of silence.

How was the week?

What went well? What else went well? And what else?

Adjust goals if necessary. What worked/didn't work? Write it here:

Mindful Life Weight Loss

The foundation of weight loss isn't the next new diet, but rather addressing the inter-relationship of the five areas that comprise a Mindful Life. Area 2 of the Five Areas of Weight Loss is food. Let's bring mindfulness to our food behavior, and to the quality of our food. There are two factors to consider: 1) our relationship with food, and 2) the quality of the food itself.

Overeating can be the result of our relationship to food. Factors such as stress, shame, fatigue, boredom, loss, loneliness, habit, proximity, misplaced desire, relationship distress, and so on, can influence eating behavior. Overeating can also be the result of the food itself. We are in a unique predicament in that our diet is filled with processed food that is designed to create craving and to override our natural signals of satiety. A diet high in processed foods alters our natural ability to regulate food intake by causing insulin and leptin resistance. (For more information on the science behind this, see the Additional Resources section at the end of this book.)

Mindful awareness will help you to determine your own unique relationship to food and your own struggles with positive food choices. Take a moment and think about your eating behavior. Think of the last time you over ate something. What did you eat? Recall what preceded the event, and what was going on in your mind, body, and environment that precipitated the eating (the trigger). Consider the type of food that you overate and investigate if it felt like it had an addictive quality to it (i.e., you can't stop after a normal amount).

Mindful Life Weight Loss

Write it down here:

The practice of mindfulness will help you to uncover what is really at the heart of your relationship with food. In the days of our ancestors, food was just food. Today, food is not just food. It is a stand-in for many things -- love, comfort, companionship, and more. Part of the benefit of mindfulness is that it will help you to uncover the role food is playing in your life and what triggers your eating behavior.

No one can discover this for you. It is something you uncover through the process of nonjudgmental awareness. As self-conscious as this process may seem, enjoy this self-discovery and approach it with a sense of curiosity and openness. You are truly at the beginning of a promising new path.

How to Choose a Diet

The first question that comes to mind when talking about weight loss is usually "what *diet* should I go on?" Atkins? Low carb? Paleo? Gluten-free? Vegan? Weight Watchers? Jenny Craig frozen meals? Mindful Life Weight Loss does not require or endorse any particular diet. Instead, we steer people away from commercialized, faddish diets.

Mindful Life Weight Loss

Don't think of this as a new diet. This is your new lifestyle. Unlike a "diet" that has a start and a finish, you will be abiding by these guidelines in one form or another for your whole life. So make sure they are guidelines you can live with.

So what should you eat? Aim for a whole foods, non-processed, non-deprivation diet. In other words, eat the majority of your food as close to its natural state as possible. Do not obsess over calories, but rather be aware of calories. Avoid overly-restrictive diets. Here are three guidelines to help you choose a diet:

1. Eat fresh, unprocessed foods.
2. Be mindful of the connection between your food choices, your body, and the planet.
3. Avoid deprivation.

1. Eat fresh, unprocessed foods. Gradually ridding your diet of refined, processed, chemically-laden food will be the most important step you take. The closer your food is to its natural state, the better. The greater the percentage of your diet that consists of these "real foods," the easier weight loss/weight maintenance will become. This cannot be overstated. How can we define unprocessed foods? These are the foods found on the periphery of the grocery store, in farmer's markets, and farm shares. They are foods as close to the Earth as possible. These foods do not have chemicals, added sugar, artificial flavorings, thickeners, additives, and preservatives. Canned or frozen foods are fine as long as they do not contain added ingredients. Avoid food with long labels, and in packages that make health claims such as "low fat!" or "heart healthy!" And seek to limit food from restaurants--especially restaurants you can drive through.

Manufactured food is designed to be hyper-palatable. It is engineered with the trinity of salt, sugar, and fat that makes you eat more than your body needs. It is enhanced with chemicals designed to blast your senses with intense flavor. It is designed -- quite deliberately -- to stimulate the same pleasure centers of the brain that are involved in addictive behaviors. When they say "You can't eat just one" they really mean it. If this makes you feel like the food industry is not your friend, then use that feeling to help you to say "no" to processed foods. The food industry employs teams of scientists, marketing experts, and psychologists to achieve one goal: for you to eat as much of their food as possible.

If this is the only change you make in your diet, you will notice an improvement. Nature did not intend for you to be in a state of hypervigilance, constantly counting calories. Nature did not intend for you to always have to be in a state of wanting more. Nature intended for you to eat nutrient-dense foods that fill you up naturally, and regulate your weight with little effort.

You may think that you don't have the time to shop for fresh food. However, this may not be the case. There are food delivery services, or community supported agriculture shares (CSAs) that can deliver food to your home. What you pay in a delivery charge might turn out to be less than eating out, or buying processed foods. There may also be a way that you can incorporate a stop at the grocery store into your daily routine, perhaps even pairing it with walking. Also, you can buy wholesome foods that are frozen, bagged, or canned to save frequent trips to the store. Be creative. This can be done if you make it a priority. Good health takes time, but poor health takes even more time.

The large, commercialized food companies (sometimes called "Big Food") want you to buy (i.e. eat) as much food as possible. They are impartial to your diabetes, obesity, heart attack risk, or general well-being. This is why-- through mindful awareness-- you must begin to care about yourself.

You can bet that if it comes in a package, or from a restaurant, it will have more sugar, fat, salt, chemicals, flavor enhancers, and calories than would be there if you cooked the food on your own.

It is time to take back control of what goes into your body, and the place to do that is in your own kitchen.

Once you make this a priority, you will find that with some planning, it will not take as much time as you think. Larger meals can be cooked in a slow-cooker while you are at work, and your family can come home to a wholesome, healthy, hot meal. Simpler meals can be "assembled" from fresh ingredients, such as salads, fruits, and a protein. You can freeze soups and stews. Tonight's dinner can be packed up for tomorrow's lunch. For me, spring through fall consists of assembled meals -- salads, sandwiches, and fresh ingredients. The cooler months consist of soups and stews cooked in large batches and frozen. Eating simple, fresh foods need not become a time-consuming activity, but it will initially require some time and planning. The rewards will be great.

2. Be mindful of the connection between your food choices, your body, and the planet. As you begin to develop the mindfulness muscle, you will expand your awareness of everything around you.

In the next chapter, you will do a mindful eating exercise inspired by Zen monk Thich Nhat Hanh's book *Savor*. As you mindfully eat an apple, you will savor the sweetness, the fruity scent, the effect it has on your body, and the cheerful beauty of the fruit. Also, you will consider all that went into creating the apple---the sunshine, air, water, farm workers, bees, birds, trucks, fuel, etc.

Every morsel of our food holds a similar story. Our eating behaviors have an effect on others. Open your awareness to this by incorporating mindful awareness of your food source. How is your food made or produced? Under what conditions? What are the consequences of the methods of production of your food? Asking yourself whether you really need as much animal-sourced food, for example, considers the great suffering farm animals endure. Buying from a local farmer, as opposed to factory/industrial agriculture is kinder to the environment, healthier, and better tasting.

Every day we hear disturbing stories of rampant safety violations, environmental degradation, and cruelty in industrial agriculture. We also hear stories of food manufacturers responding to consumer demands by going organic, featuring more vegetarian options, eliminating chemicals, and adopting more Earth-friendly practices. Your choices matter. Every dollar you spend is a vote in favor of a healthier body and a healthier planet, or the opposite.

3. Avoid deprivation. The worst thing you could do is to throw out every last box of processed food. While this might feel cathartic, in the long run, it will backfire. Deprivation only causes an internal rebellion, and creates a negative mentality. Avoid a mindset that focuses on what you are "giving up." Focus on what you are gaining. Not that you shouldn't begin clearing out the unhealthy foods--for some people with a sugar addiction, abstinence may end up being the final goal. But generally speaking, change will happen gradually and over time. And don't forget to enjoy eating. Choose only one unhealthy food to eliminate, and replace it with a healthier alternative. For example, some people start out by eliminating sugary drinks. That is far more attainable than clearing out every item that contains sugar. Over time, you may very well end up getting rid of added sugar. But not all at once.

Mindful Life in Action: What Happened When I Gave Up Processed Food

Growing up eating the standard American diet, I also grew up watching my weight. Food was something that I always wanted more of. It seemed that life was going to be a long process of wanting more, but not being able to have more. All that changed when I switched my diet away from white flour and sugar and toward unprocessed foods. After what can only be described as "sugar withdrawal," I eventually found that it was entirely possible to eat until you are full, and actually be full. The freedom of not having food on my mind was eye-opening and liberating. For years, I thought that living in a state of always wanting more food was the norm, but I realized that processed food was causing this lack of satiety. After I changed my diet, I thought "This is what food is supposed to be: fuel that you eat when you are hungry, until you are full, and don't think of it again for several hours." This was not possible when I was eating refined carbohydrates, restaurant food, and other processed food.

Setting a Food Goal

Small goals. Small changes. Allow these principles to unfold in a gradual, natural progression. Choose one of the above 3 guidelines and come up with a small, attainable food goal for the week. Examples of this might be "I will sit down to a mindful dinner three nights this week" or "I will bring my lunch to work instead of eating out this week." Write it down here.

My food goal for this week is:

I will....

Mindful Life Weight Loss

Remember that modifying your environment helps with goal success. You should set yourself up for success prior to the triggering situation, either by subtracting the problematic situations (avoiding triggers, removing foods from the home), or by adding modifications or supports (portion control, healthy food alternatives). Some examples of this are: pre-portioning out your food, removing trigger foods from the house, having healthy snack substitutes, and driving a different way home to avoid passing a food-triggering restaurant.

Mindful Life in Action: Linda Buys Flowers Instead of Ice Cream

Linda struggled with binge eating at night. She lived alone and was in a position to be in control of all the food that came into her household. Linda knew that the decisions she made at the grocery store would have a big impact on her eating behavior at home. When her favorite comfort foods were not in the house, she would go to sleep earlier rather than stay up late eating. One day when Linda was grocery shopping she made a pivotal decision. When faced with buying ice cream, her favorite comfort food, she chose a beautiful bouquet of flowers instead. Flowers symbolized Linda's self-love and desire to be healthy and happy. When evening came and her resolve was low, she did not have problematic foods around. Instead, she had the flowers reminding her of her commitment to herself.

Mindful Life Weight Loss

Increasing accountability involves building in checkpoints. Goals that are made privately to ourselves are weak goals. You will need to "go public" by enlisting at least one other person. Perhaps you can join an online dieting community where you post our food goals each day, enlist the help of a friend or family member, work with a trainer or coach, or make your goals public on social media. Goals that have built-in accountability are more likely to be goals that are attained.

Some ways I will modify my environment to achieve this goal are:

Some ways I will increase my accountability to achieve this goal are:

Hunger, Craving, and Desire *(with credit to Jan Chozen Bays' book *Mindful Eating*)

Hunger is your body's signal that it is time to eat. This is natural and good. However, many people experience the physical sensation of hunger and view it as a state of emergency, and respond in an out-of-proportion way. While we should heed our body's signals, normal everyday hunger is not an emergency. Most people eating a standard American diet are very far removed from their natural signals of hunger and satiety—processed food interferes with feelings of normal hunger. Once you move toward natural, simpler foods, you will gain a better idea of what normal hunger feels like.

Mindfully examine what feelings arise when confronted with hunger in order to gain a better understanding of how you handle this physical sensation. Mindfulness practice will help you to develop "distress tolerance" in small doses, so you are better prepared to respond to normal hunger.

Excessive hunger will cause you to overeat and skipping meals will also trigger overeating, so try to structure your meals/snacks in a way to avoid feeling too hungry, while allowing yourself to feel moderate hunger. A good rule of thumb is to have three meals a day, and two nutritious snacks between meals if needed. Some people do fine with three meals, while others need to have a few snacks. Listen to your body.

When you are feeling the sensation of hunger, take ten mindful breaths to examine your internal state. After the ten breaths, you will probably have a better idea of whether you are feeling genuine hunger, boredom, stress, thirst, tiredness, or another sensation. Also, what you think is hunger may actually be craving or desire.

Craving is often the result of a junk-food addiction, or a chronically unhealthy diet. The food industry deliberately manufactures food to produce craving and dependency. If you eat a processed food diet, much of what you perceive as hunger is probably craving. Rarely do we crave an apple or some almonds. People don't usually lament on how they are unable to have just one broccoli spear, or drive out at midnight to pick up a bag of sweet potatoes. Usually, we crave chips, ice cream, or a fast food---foods that have been specifically created to produce cravings. Over-reliance on these foods may also cause deficiencies in nutrients that present themselves as cravings.

Think of how the word "craving" has evolved in our cultural vocabulary. These days, people speak of "craving" quite frequently. A few generations ago when people ate whole foods, and food marketing wasn't rampant, this was not the case. Cravings can also be sparked by television advertisements, environmental cues, or social settings.

The good news is that slowly, over time, you can restructure your lifestyle so that you are not controlled by cravings. Many people report that cravings disappear entirely when they eat a nutrient-dense, whole foods diet. In the meantime, use nonjudgmental awareness to become aware of your cravings and potential triggers. For now, begin noticing without judgment, and come from a place of self-care.

Desire to eat can be caused by several things: simple habit; an emotional trigger; a social ritual; a holiday; using food as a reward; viewing an appealing food advertisement; and so on. And sometimes we simply want a certain food for no other reason than that we enjoy it.

Mindful Life Weight Loss

It is important to gain clarity of what lies behind the desire to eat. That way you can make intentional decisions that are in line with your goals. This may be one of the more tricky areas to address, and will require the tools of mindful awareness, self-compassion, and patience. Next time you have the desire to eat, take ten mindful breaths and see what your inner wisdom says you really want.

Knowing that you are eating out of desire, rather than necessity, can give you a greater sense of control over your behavior. The decision becomes yours, rather than unconscious habit.

ACTION STEPS:

NEXT TIME YOU EAT, ASK YOURSELF IF YOU ARE EATING OUT OF HUNGER, CRAVING, OR DESIRE.

KEEP A FOOD DIARY. TRY TO IDENTIFY WHETHER YOUR EATING BEHAVIOR STEMMED FROM HUNGER, CRAVING, OR A DESIRE TO EAT.

REWRITE YOUR FOOD GOAL HERE:

I WILL:

ADD YOUR NEW GOAL TO YOUR VISION STATEMENT, AND ACHIEVE THAT GOAL THIS WEEK. REMEMBER TO CONTINUE WITH YOUR HABIT CHANGE GOAL AS WELL!

5

Mindful Eating

> IF YOU TRULY GET IN TOUCH WITH A PIECE OF CARROT, YOU GET IN TOUCH WITH THE SOIL, THE RAIN, THE SUNSHINE. YOU GET IN TOUCH WITH MOTHER EARTH AND EATING IN SUCH A WAY, YOU FEEL IN TOUCH WITH TRUE LIFE, YOUR ROOTS, AND THAT IS MEDITATION. IF WE CHEW EVERY MORSEL OF OUR FOOD IN THAT WAY WE BECOME GRATEFUL AND WHEN YOU ARE GRATEFUL, YOU ARE HAPPY.
> THICH NHAT HANH

Begin with three minutes of silence.

How was the week?

What went well? How did you accomplish that?

How were the goals you set for yourself surrounding habits and food?

Mindful Life Weight Loss

What worked/didn't work?

What can be adjusted or changed?

Did you keep a food diary? If not, what got in the way?

What did you discover?

We have learned the basics of mindfulness, as well as the components of a healthy diet. Now it is time to focus on putting these together and practicing mindful eating.

Our taste buds and sensibilities have been conditioned to expect a cacophony of flavor, texture, and sensation. And then we continue to expect and demand more. Going down this path has not served us well, as we become desensitized to flavor. Like a drug addict, we will always need more to achieve the same effect.

Try to bring some of this mindful attention into your daily eating. Mindful eating can help you to see food in a new way. Modern food is engineered to overwhelm the senses with hyper-palatable foods, and to create craving.

Mindful Life Weight Loss

Take an apple, or another piece of fruit. Take ten mindful breaths and center yourself in the present moment. Now, using the following sample mindful eating exercise, try to eat the apple mindfully.

Here's a sample mindful eating meditation to get you started.

Hold the apple in your hand. Notice its color, various shades of red, flecks of green, its shine. Pick it up in your hand and take a few breaths. Feel its solidity and appreciate its beauty. Does it have a stem on it? Perhaps a leaf is still attached? Consider the tree it came from. If it is seasonal, perhaps it came from a local orchard in your same state. If not, consider where the apple traveled from. Think about all the people who were involved in bringing the apple from seed to maturity; the farmer, the farm workers, the truck drivers, store owners, cashiers. Reflect on the elements of nature that brought you the apple; the sun, rain, insects, animals, and our dependence on them. Think about how fortunate you are to have this apple, and that insects, excessive frost or rain did not destroy the tree.

Take a moment of gratitude for everything that has brought the apple to your hand, and for a body that can enjoy it. A miracle. Now, take a bite. Feel the crisp moisture, notice if the apple is sweet or tart. Feel its texture in your mouth. Enjoy the flavor and the aroma. Notice differences in flavor and texture from bite to bite. Eat slowly, and let the flavor fill your being. Notice how your body feels as it responds to the apple. Is this different from processed food? How?

Mindful Life Weight Loss

Notice the thoughts that go through your own mind, without judgment...Continue eating the apple in this manner.

Of course, each person's mindful eating experience will be different. Once the above exercise gets you started, follow your mind and see where the meditation leads you.

Mindful Life in Action: Eating on a Zen Retreat

My first Zen meditation retreat was a total surprise for me. I signed up for it, thinking that it would be a relaxing three days away from my busy life. However, I soon learned that a Zen retreat is very disciplined and structured. Conducted entirely in silence, we spent about 8 hours of the day in seated meditation. We had brief periods of walking meditation, and three meals. These meals were considered part of meditation. We were instructed to be fully present with every aspect of the meal. Everything from the way we drank tea, to how deliberately our forks met the plate, to how many times we chewed was with full presence of mind and body. The heightened attention had the effect of making the simple food some of the most memorable and tasty food I have ever experienced. Eating mindfully was at once sublime, sacred, and entirely ordinary. The long periods of meditation allowed my mind to settle. Without the usual mental chatter cluttering up my mind, eating was a full sensory experience: everything felt heightened. I'm sure

Mindful Life Weight Loss

the retreat center did not have access to especially tasty food, more brightly colored fruit, and crisper vegetables. It was my state of mind--my mindful presence--that amplified the experience. I learned that this state of mind can be accessed any time, for eating and other ordinary activities as well.

Consider your experience with eating the apple. This piece of fruit was not engineered in a lab. The apple tree has no vested interest in whether or not you buy more apples, so it is not modified to create craving. This is real food. When the mind is quiet and free from artificial distractions, an apple can be a sublime experience. Its sweetness, crispness, and nutrients can fill up body, mind, and spirit. You don't always need apple pie, sticky gooey cinnamon apple donuts, or apple crisp. The apple contains the whole world, and an enticing bouquet of flavor and texture. Mindful eating entails learning to savor each bite of food. Mindful eating is a central component to your daily mindfulness practice.

What were three things you discovered while doing the mindful eating exercise:

1.

2.

3.

Mindful Life Weight Loss

How did this compare with the way you usually eat?

Mindfulness is a practical skill that is designed to fit into our real-world lives. People are not likely to sound a mindfulness bell and eat this way every meal. We are not monks and nuns. However, it is possible to invite more mindfulness into your everyday eating behavior. Not only will you make healthier choices, but you may find that you enjoy your food more.

Here are five ways to bring mindfulness into everyday eating:

1. *When you eat, eat.* An old Zen adage can be loosely paraphrased as follows: When you walk, walk. When you chop wood, chop wood. When you boil rice, boil rice. As much as possible, try to avoid eating while doing other tasks. It is easy to lose track of how much you eat and your body's natural signals if you are engrossed in a television show or work project.

Mealtime will "stretch to fit" whatever activity you are pairing it with. If you simply stop what you are doing to eat, you will be less motivated to extend your eating past what is necessary. Perhaps you will even be more motivated to stop eating sooner so you can resume that interesting project or show. You are also more likely to savor and enjoy your food if it is the only thing you are doing.

2. *Buy the best quality food you can afford, even if you buy less of it.* With an awareness of where our food comes from, begin to take small steps to buy organic, fair trade, local, seasonal, humane, non-

Mindful Life Weight Loss

GMO, or whatever you define as "best quality" foods, whenever possible.

Yes, that container of organic strawberries is more expensive than the conventional version. However, when you eat them you can really savor them---admire their rich redness, natural sweetness, and wholesomeness. You will know that the farmer did not have to don a Hazmat suit to spray them with pesticides. Good quality food tastes better.

You will also be more inclined to eat food that is closer to its natural state when you shop with this awareness. Rather than bury the anemic strawberries under sugar and whipped cream (and calories), over time you will begin to appreciate their simple beauty and flavor, and maybe make an event of eating them as is.

3. *Eat as a family*. While studies show that we tend to eat more when we are in groups, studies also show many more benefits to family mealtime (improved grades, reduction in childhood obesity, improved behavior in children). The benefits of eating together clearly outweigh the small risk that you may eat more---especially if you are serving healthy food and eating without the television or computer. Humans have been eating in groups for as long as we can remember, yet obesity is a recent phenomenon. The tendency to eat alone in front of our screens contributes to our increasing isolation from each other. This isolation leads to stress, loneliness, and emotional eating to compensate for the emptiness of modern life. Leading a Mindful Life means mindfully

tending to our whole lives, and the contexts in which we eat.

4. *Set the table with real dishes and sit down.* Sometimes we have to eat on the run. And sometimes we eat take-out. But if we begin to live more intentionally, those can be the exceptions rather than the rule.

When you eat on real dishes instead of takeout containers, you can better control your portion size. Normal-sized dinner plates are far different from the portion that comes in a take-out container (which might really be two or three portions). They are a far cry from the platter-sized plates that restaurants use.

Also, real tableware has a way of conveying the message that you have had a real meal. What you eat on disposable plastic or paper doesn't feel as worthy of respect, and you might not register it as "dinner" and be more likely to eat more later.

Your life simply doesn't allow for this? No problem. Remember: think small and attainable. Find one meal in your entire week where you can have a real, old-school, sit-down dinner. See how that goes.

5. *Make eating a priority.* When you sit down to a meal, your mind and body register that you have eaten a legitimate meal. When you eat a fast food burger in the car on the way to take the kids to practice, your body does not think "meal" and you are more likely to eat more than you should during the rest of the day. You are likely to classify food on the

Mindful Life Weight Loss

run as "not really eating." This is also true when people eat standing up, in the car, or while working. When you deliberately, intentionally make healthy eating important, your body will check off the official "ate a meal" box and you will be less likely to compensate by overeating later.

If your meals are currently not a priority, it is worth asking why. What else is a priority? What are the consequences of that?

Action steps:

Enjoy a mindful, undistracted meal of wholesome ingredients with your family or a friend this week. Notice what arose for you. Consider the following questions and record your answers here:

Did you enjoy your food more?

Did you eat less? Did you get hungry later?

What other effects did you notice?

Were any other areas of your life affected by this one change?

Mindful Life Weight Loss

Remember to keep your Vision Statement, with your two goals, posted in prominent places.

6

Born to Move

> **MINDFULNESS HELPS YOU GO HOME TO THE PRESENT. AND EVERY TIME YOU GO THERE AND RECOGNIZE A CONDITION OF HAPPINESS THAT YOU HAVE, HAPPINESS COMES.**
> **THICH NHAT HANH**

Begin with three minutes of silence.

How was the week?

What went well?

How was your mindful meal homework?

What worked/didn't work?

What can be adjusted or changed?

Mindful Life Weight Loss

How are the other habits and goals coming along (refer to Vision Statement)?

What has been the effect of some of these small changes on your weight? You don't want to become overly-focused on a number on the scale, but the number is a useful guide for you.

Now that you are several steps along on your path, have you had any unexpected changes? Is it harder or easier than you originally thought it would be?

Moving more and sitting less will most certainly improve your health, energy, vitality, and aid in your weight loss effort. Area Three of the Five Areas of Weight Loss focuses on exercise and movement. Exercise and movement are both integral parts of a Mindful Life.

While exercise and movement each play an important part in a Mindful Life, they are not synonymous. Exercise is any activity that requires physical effort done to improve strength or fitness, i.e. a sport, brisk walking, jogging, lifting weights, yoga, etc.

Movement, for the purposes of this program, is defined as anything other than sitting.

There is no need to embark upon a radical exercise plan. Small, incremental changes are a long-term path to permanent change.

Mindful Life Weight Loss

If you are not at a point in your life where you want to embrace an exercise regimen, you can start by increasing movement. You will find that an increase in movement will produce surprising changes in your energy and health. If you would like to do more vigorous exercise, that is great too—we'll discuss that more in the next chapter.

Movement can encompass standing at your computer workstation, shopping, cooking, cleaning house, light chores, waiting in line, or leisurely walking. A good way to measure movement is to wear a pedometer or portable fitness tracker.

Most people grossly over-estimate their movement, and are shocked to find out how little they move when they look at a pedometer. Most people are also shocked to learn how much activity is required to burn off the calories found in their everyday diet.

Mindful Life in Action: How I Fit Movement into an Impossible Schedule

Back in 2005, my husband was quite sick. He needed major surgery, and a long recovery period. Our children were both small, and my days were jam packed with caring for small children and driving back and forth to the hospital. I knew, however, that I needed to do something to keep my body moving to help manage the stress. Sitting around the hospital and long trips in the car only made the stress worse. Yet it seemed impossible to exercise with all I had going on. I decided to buy a pedometer and focus on footsteps rather than getting a workout. Activity rather than exercise. In doing this, I was able to take walks up and down the hospital corridor, up stairs, around the block, and other small trips to add up to thousands of steps per day. This helped me to clear my head and relax, and proved to me that if I could fit movement into my life during this time, then I can do it any time.

As with the other areas of the program, the first step to changing your habits is mindfulness. Think for a moment about your daily habits surrounding movement. Become aware of how much time you spend sitting and lying down, how you unwind and relax, how much television you watch, how your body feels after a long day of sitting at the office, etc. Become aware of your attitudes and beliefs about movement and exercise.

Some questions to consider are:

Do you work on your feet or sitting down?

Do you take the stairs?

Do you walk anywhere?

How much housework do you normally do?

Do you lift or bend as part of your daily routine?

Do you do any outdoor chores (shoveling, raking, gardening)?

Do you have any health conditions or injuries that limit your activity?

There are countless studies that show that excessive sitting--or sedentary behavior--is a major health risk. The saying "Sitting is the new smoking" is not far from the truth.

Overall mortality, as well as specific diseases such as cancer and heart disease are increased by something as seemingly innocuous as sitting. Additionally, children who are deprived of outdoor playtime have difficulties learning and concentrating. If you bring your mindful attention to how your body and mind feels after a day of sitting, you will probably notice that you don't feel very good at all.

From an evolutionary perspective, our bodies are meant to move. Since the dawn of human history, we have been on the go, walking long distances, lifting heavy objects, bending, and standing. It wasn't until fairly recently---just a few generations---that we began to increase the amount of time that we spend sitting down. In fact, much of our modern lifestyle seems to require a seated position.

We are contrasting the entirety of human history with just a couple of generations when it comes to changing our movement habits. Look where it has gotten us. If you ask most people how they feel, you will likely get an answer that reflects poor health.

Obviously, we cannot go back to a time when we walked miles to the nearest watering hole and carried the water home on our backs. What we can do is increase the amount of movement in our lives--- breaking up our blocks of sedentary time, changing the way we do our chores, adding a few hundred steps here and there. This will have an effect. Remember that systems thinking does not require large sweeping changes, but states that small changes in one area can have significant results. The ripple effect is a powerful phenomenon. Think in terms of footsteps, not miles.

Mindful Life in Action: Erica and the Stairs

Erica has a very busy job in publishing in New York City. Her commute from the suburbs means that she leaves very early and returns home late. She rarely has time to exercise, but she didn't want to let that stop her from being healthy. Her one small goal was to always take the stairs when she needed to go three stories or less. Always. No matter how much of a rush she was in. Over time, it really added up. She used to be winded at the top of each flight, but then it became effortless and a completely natural part of her lifestyle. Additionally, her kids picked up the same habit. Erica didn't stop with the stairs (because small changes lead to big results). She downloaded an activity tracker on her phone and started to add footsteps to her day. Her goal was 10,000 and she frequently met this goal walking to and from Grand Central Station, and taking walking breaks from her daily work tasks.

Here are three tips to add some basic movement into your day:

1. Use technology-based tools to increase movement. Consider one of the devices that track footsteps, like Erica did. Some of these devices will even vibrate every 20 minutes or so to remind you to get up and walk around. Additionally, these devices tap into the human tendency to want to challenge or improve what we have done. If you find yourself walking 1,000 steps one day, try to get to 1,100 the next day. And so on.
2. Do it yourself (DIY). Look at your routine and find one task that you normally automate or outsource. Perhaps your entire family could embark upon a group housecleaning on the weekend. Have you become accustomed to asking others to do things for you because it is too tiring? Try doing a little more yourself. Do you use a machine to blow away your leaves? Perhaps your family could rake once a week. Have you gotten in the habit of ordering groceries from a delivery service or household items from Amazon Prime? Why should the UPS guy get all the exercise? Take back some of those tasks and go to the brick and mortar stores. Rake, shovel, sweep, lift, bend, push. Use the tool of mindfulness to turn the task into a family activity, or an opportunity for couple/social time, or maybe put on your headphones and listen to some music while vacuuming. Use some of the behavioral tools of reinforcement to take the money you save

and reward yourself with something desirable (but not food-related).
3. Connect. Our lives have gotten very isolated and sedentary, and it has become the new normal. Being isolated and being sedentary are linked. Consider this: we stay in our homes while products get delivered. The kids sit in front of the TV while we put the groceries away. We sit in the car and use drive-thru windows. Some of us rarely get outside in our own backyards because the family is scattered at their own activities or work. We get "curb side" pick-ups at restaurants. Too many people eat alone in their cars. Our kids stay strapped in strollers because it is easier than chasing them around. Teens don't even physically get together anymore, as kids text and face time as a form of social interaction. Simply making an effort to connect with other flesh and blood human beings will increase movement as we go places and do things. This ripple effect will lead to more movement (akin to what earlier generations experienced) and decreased isolation.

People have a tendency to over-estimate how much they move and how many calories are burned with any given activity. We will talk more next chapter about calories and exercise. Combining a modest but consistent increase in movement with more mindful eating habits can take you very far in your weight loss goals.

Mindful Life Weight Loss

Mindful awareness is always the first step, and half the battle. This week we are simply going to understand what our baseline is, and take a small step to improve that.

Let's consider our habits surrounding movement that we talked about earlier. Look at a typical day and identify three areas where you could move more. Perhaps you can take a few more steps, go up an extra flight of stairs, park a little farther from the building, rake the leaves yourself, walk somewhere instead of drive, take the dog for a walk rather than letting him outside, play catch with your kid, etc. Think small and manageable. Additionally, if you are curious about your level of movement, try a pedometer or fitness tracker.

Write down one way that you could increase your daily movement:

1.

Next, formulate a specific goal targeting this habit, and write it on your Vision Statement.

Goals should be small, attainable, measurable, and accountable.

MY GOAL:

I will....

Mindful Life Weight Loss

List the way (or ways) that I will be accountable for this goal:

List how you can set up your environment for success regarding this goal:

ACTION STEPS:

ATTAIN THE GOAL THAT YOU HAVE SET FOR YOURSELF REGARDING INCREASING YOUR DAILY MOVEMENT. ADD IT TO YOUR VISION STATEMENT. YOU NOW HAVE MANY TOOLS IN YOUR TOOLKIT TO HELP YOU WITH THIS.

REWRITE YOUR ACTIVITY GOAL HERE.

I WILL...

ALSO REMEMBER YOUR GOALS ABOUT HABITS AND FOOD. YOU NOW HAVE THREE SMALL GOALS WORKING SIMULTANEOUSLY, SO KEEP YOUR VISION STATEMENT POSTED IN PLACES WHERE YOU CAN SEE IT. SOON, IF YOU KEEP IT UP, THOSE GOALS WILL BECOME NEW HABITS THAT ARE AS INGRAINED AS YOUR OLD HABITS. KEEP IT UP!

7

Effortless Exercise

YOU CAN'T OUT-RUN A BAD DIET.
AUTHOR UNKNOWN

Begin with three minutes of silence.

How did last week's movement goal go?

What went well?

What did not work? For problematic times, how were you able to prevent the problems from becoming even worse than they could have been?

Check in with your habit goal and food goal.

What areas of your life are better this week?

As we discussed in the last chapter, exercise is an activity done to build strength and improve fitness. It is different from basic movement.

Our ancestors did not have to exercise. The daily activities of life were rigorous enough to maintain fitness without adding any additional movement. Can you imagine a woman who routinely carried large jugs of water for miles coming home and lifting barbells? Or imagine a man who ran miles hunting an animal needing to run on a treadmill? Even the very concept of modern exercise equipment seems strange in light of the functional purpose of our bodies (a $500 machine that allows you to run to nowhere?).

Our modern-day habits are a major deviation from what our bodies have done since the beginning of human history. But then again, so are our diets and lifestyles. Indeed, what we call "exercise" in modern times is merely a re-creation of what our bodies were designed to do: run, jump, lift, and bend.

While we might have a few years, or decades, of sedentary habits, humanity as a whole has far more momentum in the direction of movement. This should inspire hope.

You have all of human history pulling for you!

Sadly, for many of us, exercise is perceived as an unpleasant medicine. Something to be done as little as possible, and only when necessary. For others, exercise may in fact be fun, but the demands and habits of everyday life crowd it out of our schedules.

Mindful Life Weight Loss

Just like food, exercise has context. What comes to mind when the word "exercise" is mentioned? Take a moment to bring your mindful attention to your thoughts and feelings about exercise. Complete the following sentence:

When I think of exercise, I feel..

Last time I tried an exercise program, I...

One thing that would make me really want to exercise is................................

One thing that keeps me from exercising is..

Wherever you fall on the spectrum---probably somewhere in between the extremes---we are going to examine why and how to re-introduce exercise into our lifestyle.

The Benefits of Exercise

Let's begin by remembering why exercise is so vital. It seems that every day there is a new study about the benefits of exercise. If the pharmaceutical companies could create a drug that did all of these things and had almost zero side-effects...imagine.

Exercise ...

improves muscle tone
improves mood
lowers blood pressure
increases bone density
improves mental acuity
lowers cholesterol
reduces stress
improves sex drive
protects against Alzheimer's disease
protects against cancer
improves sleep
burns calories
keeps you feeling young
regulates appetite
increases longevity
increases stamina
improves energy
helps with depression (it is an evidence-based intervention for depression)
and can be fun!

It also seems that there is a new form of exercise program coming out every year---Zumba, Crossfit, spinning...the list goes on. This is good news. When it comes to exercise, there is something for everyone.

If you have had bad experiences with exercise in the past, it is simply because you haven't found the right one (or the right instructor, class, sport, etc.)—so don't give up.

To some of you this may sound far-fetched, but it's true: Exercise can and should be fun. If exercise is

Mindful Life Weight Loss

fun and engaging, you will be more likely to make it into a habit. Life is too short to endure a torturous workout that you hate.

Mindful Life in Action: Leslie's Spin Class that Couldn't Be Missed

Leslie had found her effortless exercise. She loved a particular spin class that combined exercise, great music, and motivational quotes. Leslie was introduced to these classes while visiting a friend who lived about 45 minutes away. However, Leslie could not find a spin studio similar to this one in her own town. So, even though Leslie had a very busy schedule, she found a way to make it to these classes at least once per week. She did not mind the long drive, and didn't even let the snow keep her away. Leslie would often come to our groups and describe these classes as her personal form of therapy and stress relief. She exclaimed "This is how exercise should be: the highlight of my week."

Here are five tips to consider when looking for an enjoyable form of exercise:

1. *Choose a "just right" activity.* Be selective about which program you choose. When you observe or try a class, how do you feel? Intimidated? Insecure? Made to push beyond what you feel is safe? Bored? Excited? Invigorated? Trust your inner voice. If your gut is saying "no," then listen. First impressions

matter. There are plenty of choices out there. Give yourself permission to walk away if it is not the right fit. Don't force yourself to start the wrong regimen because you think you must. That will only create negative momentum when you inevitably quit. Just say "no" to one thing, so that you can say "yes" to something better. Once you find something you truly enjoy, motivation will come easily.

2. *Know thyself.* It was true for the ancient Greeks, and it is true today. Knowing what type of person you are will help you choose an activity that lasts. Personality should match activity. Are you an introvert? Well, then it is no wonder you don't enjoy a team sport, or a noisy spin class. Are you an extrovert? Perhaps a quiet yoga class is not for you. Do you prefer to compete with yourself or others? Do you like the challenge of a steep learning curve, or do you like to "get it" right way? Are you looking for a lifelong practice (a martial art, yoga) or do you like to try new things? Do you get bored easily? Do you like the outdoors? Hate the outdoors? And so on. Many people quit an exercise regimen because it wasn't a good fit for their personality. Factoring this in at the beginning improves your chances of finding something you will stick with.

3. *Choose realistic activities.* Take an honest look at your whole life. If you suddenly decide that swimming will be your exercise of choice, can you realistically say that you can get to the indoor pool on a regular basis? Schedule time to change, shower, commute? Can you afford the gear or fees required for the activity you choose? Can your work schedule accommodate the exercise class schedule? Are you

relying on a partner to work out with? Is that partner reliable? Do you have any physical limitations that will interfere with this type of exercise? For example, if you have bad knees, running might not be realistic. Many exercise intentions fail because they were unrealistic choices given a person's lifestyle, budget, work schedule, or body type. Improve your chances of success by getting real in the beginning.

4. *Look for built-in accountability.* This is most important in the beginning stages of forming a habit. Seasoned exercisers don't need this as much, as working out becomes second nature. The morning run is as habituated as the morning coffee.

Beginners need built-in accountability---the training wheels of habit formation. An activity that relies entirely on your own willpower is not likely to succeed. The force of habit is too strong, and willpower is notoriously fluctuating and unreliable. Vowing to do the 30-minute YouTube kettle bell workout three times a week is not likely to stick. Sure, you may say, "it is free, easy, and convenient." However, it is also unlikely to become your new habit.

Rather, look for activities that have some kind of built-in accountability in the beginning. Work with a trainer for the first couple of months of your gym membership, join a yoga school and become part of the community, take up a martial art and get to know your training partners, join a running or walking club, pair up with a friend, hire a coach, sign up and pre-pay for a block of classes, etc. You can do that free YouTube workout, but do it with a group or friend.

Mindful Life Weight Loss

Additionally, to increase accountability, share your exercise goals with your weight loss group, coach, or partners. Let the group know that you plan to go to a Zumba class two times this week, and ask someone to check in by text to keep you honest. Feel free to use the Mindful Life Weight Loss Facebook page for support. If you post your goals and intentions, the group will keep you accountable and supported.

Use the power of relationship to aid in your accountability.

5. *And finally, have fun!* Exercise should be fun. No pain, no gain is outdated. To quote YouTube yogi Adrienne, from Yoga with Adrienne: "Find what feels good."

Sometimes exercise pushes you, is uncomfortable, and you are sore the next day. But fun is found in the big picture, not in the particulars. Overall, do you feel better or worse? Did you smile at all?

Exercise should be an overall positive experience, even if you have sore hamstrings the next day. If it is not fun, find something else to do that is!

If you keep these five things in mind, you should be able to find the right fit when it comes to working out.

Mindful Life in Action: The Day I Started Martial Arts

I was 38 years old and had spent far too many years on the treadmill. I actually wore out a treadmill after about a decade, and had to get a new one. When the new treadmill was destroyed in a basement flood, I took it as divine guidance that I should find a form of exercise that was truly fun and engaging. Running to nowhere was, well, getting me nowhere. I'm not completely discounting it, as it served me well for many years. It was a great stress reliever, cardiovascular workout, and it helped me to clear my head. But I wanted something more. Something that I could learn and eventually master. Something that was exciting as well as practical. And something that challenged me and pushed my limits. I found that in the martial art of Aikido, a bit late in life, but better late than never. Making sure I attended practice was effortless, because I loved every minute of it. I loved the mental discipline, spirituality, beauty, and challenge of it. I was disappointed if something got in the way of my workout. It is a true gift to be able to have an "effortless exercise" in my life, as I never consider it a chore and don't have to work to fit it into my schedule.

But, What About Burning Calories?

It is true that exercise burns calories. Everything burns calories to some extent. However, burning calories should not be the primary reason to exercise. Exercise is going to have to be a permanent part of your lifestyle, not just what you do when you want to burn off something you ate. You will need to change your relationship to exercise from a few dates to a happy marriage. Just like you are not "going on a diet" to lose weight (because diets don't work), you are not "exercising to lose weight." You will need to find an exercise program and frequency that you can stick with over the course of your lifetime. In order to do this you will actually have to derive pleasure from the activity, or you will quickly lose motivation. "Burning calories" is simply not enough motivation to sustain a lifestyle that includes exercise.

Additionally, you really can't out-run a bad diet. If you are eating a diet filled with high-calorie, processed foods, it is unlikely that you will be able to do enough exercise to keep a healthy weight. You'd have to do an extreme amount of exercise to out-run a Big Mac-- and even then the health problems would still catch up with you. If you are among the metabolically blessed who never gains an ounce, a bad diet will harm your health in many other ways. Weight loss really does begin in the kitchen, and exercise should be a part of your life for the myriad health benefits besides burning calories.

Body Awareness: A Useful Side Effect of Exercise

Let's face it: we live in our heads. Our bodies are merely the vehicle to carry our minds around from place to place. And with so much being automated, we don't really even use our body to go very far. Living in our heads has many problems. We are cut off from what happens in our body, and we frequently bypass or ignore its messages. We are not in touch with our bodily signals. We cannot truly feel the effect of stress or sleep deprivation, and we drive our bodies like a cruel taskmaster. We do not notice the effect of sugar and processed food on our moods and digestion. We do not sense when we are overeating, or depriving ourselves of vital nutrients. We often lose sight of cause and effect relationships between our behavior and our bodies.

Exercise---especially mindfulness-based exercise---brings us out of our heads and into our bodies. A frequent admonition in yoga classes is "listen to your body." And indeed, one of yoga's main benefits is that it improves body awareness. Mindfulness of the body is a key skill in weight loss. Once you get used to listening to and responding to your body, you are solidly on the path of lifelong weight loss. Your body has all the wisdom it needs to direct you toward healthy food, activity, and behaviors. Listen to it.

Mindful Life in Action: Susan's Swimming Teaches Her to Listen to Her Body

Susan began the Mindful Life program after decades of inactivity. She was recently retired, and worked part-time. She could not remember the last time she exercised. Several of Susan's group sessions focused on finding an exercise that would be fun, and also safe for her bad knees. She decided to go to the pool in her apartment complex, not as a form of "exercise" but rather as a way to enjoy the warm summer days. Susan focused on simply enjoying herself in the water. She began to do her own spontaneous version of a water workout--bobbing up and down, treading water, and light swimming. She remarked that she felt a sense of joy and ease when she was in the pool. She structured her day around her pool sessions. She also noticed that she was able to tune into

Mindful Life Weight Loss

her body more easily at other times. She was eating differently---stopping when she was full, choosing lighter foods, and had not binged at all. Susan's somatic awareness in the pool had carried over to other parts of her life. Susan was re-learning how to listen to her body.

ACTION STEPS:

THIS WEEK, BEGIN AN EXPLORATION PROCESS SURROUNDING EXERCISE. SEARCH AROUND THE INTERNET, YOU TUBE, LOCAL GYMS, AND SEE WHAT APPEALS TO YOU. USE YOUR MINDFUL AWARENESS TO CONSIDER THE ABOVE-MENTIONED TIPS. NARROW DOWN THE FIELD TO THREE FORMS OF EXERCISE THAT INTRIGUE YOU.

LIST THEM HERE:

1.

2.

3.

OVER THE NEXT FEW WEEKS, BEGIN TO EXPLORE BY OBSERVING CLASSES, TRYING CLASSES, OR SPEAKING TO OTHERS ABOUT YOUR CHOICES. DON'T SETTLE UNTIL YOU FIND SOMETHING THAT YOU LOVE.

8

Thinking in Systems

> WHATEVER AFFECTS ONE DIRECTLY, AFFECTS ALL INDIRECTLY. I CAN NEVER BE WHAT I OUGHT TO BE UNTIL YOU ARE WHAT YOU OUGHT TO BE. THIS IS THE INTERRELATED STRUCTURE OF REALITY.
> MARTIN LUTHER KING, JR.

Begin with three minutes of silence.

How did the week go?

How was your exploration in exercise? What did you come up with?

What went well?

What did not work/needs to be adjusted?

How are your other goals going (refer to Vision Statement)?

Mindful Life Weight Loss

For many of you, one week of experimenting did not yield an exercise activity that you want to pursue. That is okay. Don't give up on exercising, but know that you can still lose weight if you follow the other parts of the plan while you continue your search for an enjoyable form of exercise. The basics of systems thinking will help to understand why.

Systems thinking is a useful paradigm to understand the multiple causes and contexts of the behaviors that comprise a weight loss program. Systems theory is a way of looking at the world that sees things in terms of the whole picture rather than isolated parts, or just the sum of its parts. Looking at things this way is called "relational thinking." Systems theory sees things from multiple perspectives, not just one. Thus, it provides multiple solutions and creative problem solving. Systems thinking contains a useful technology that shows us the most effective leverage points to create the most change for the least amount of effort.

Systems thinking has a very broad reach and been applied to many fields including sociology, psychology, biology, engineering, philosophy, and many others. It has its origins with Austrian biologist Ludwig Von Bertalanffy in the 1930s, and from there was adapted by thinkers from disparate fields. I was introduced to systems thinking while studying for my M.S. in Marriage and Family Therapy (MFT). Many of the models of human behavior in the MFT field are based on systems thinking. Most MFTs are trained to be systems thinkers and see interrelationships.

Mindful Life Weight Loss

Mindful Life in Action: Addressing Laura's Binge Eating

Laura was a 55 year old woman who lived alone, and worked an evening shift that ended at 10 pm. She would stay up very late into the night eating out of loneliness. These binges used to end at around midnight, but over time they expanded to as late at 4 a.m. Laura would read, surf the web, or watch TV while eating. Her life had been turned literally upside down as she was now eating alone in her apartment all night, and sleeping most of the day. Further, in order to not gain weight, Laura ate very little food other than during her binges, leaving her ravenously hungry by 10 pm. Laura came into our program because she needed to change something, but was afraid of giving up the comforting behavior of binge eating. She had tried psychotherapy, dietitians, Overeaters Anonymous, and other programs. Each program wanted to address the binge eating, which was a terrifying concept for Laura, as for many binge eaters. She asked if I could help her take small steps, and not start with the binges. As a systems thinker, I understand that there is more than one entry point to a problem, so I said yes. Laura came up with the idea of gradually normalizing her sleep schedule. I worked with Laura to wake up incrementally earlier and earlier, until she had normalized her sleep schedule. Then, Laura began eating three meals a day-- something she never thought she would be able to do. She noticed that when she was not starving, her binges were a small fraction of what they once were. They were on their way out. We also made the observation that the middle of the night is a lonely time for anyone, and Laura was able to be more engaged with life during the daylight hours. Her loneliness subsided somewhat. Laura's was able to address

Mindful Life Weight Loss

one problematic area of her life by making changes in another seemingly unrelated area. That is systems thinking.

Your lifestyle can be considered a "system." A system is defined as an entity comprised of parts that operate in relationship to each other. These parts produce a "whole" that is your lifestyle. Your life cannot simply be reduced to the sum of its parts. Most weight loss programs try to do this by reducing weight loss to diet or exercise. However, diet and exercise cannot be taken out of context, and must be viewed in relationship to all of the parts of your life. In Laura's case, addressing diet was counterproductive, but addressing another area--sleep---proved to be the most effective entry point. Like Laura, everyone's problems have multiple entry points.

A Broken System

This has likely happened to you before: You go on a diet, and you lose the weight. Then, you gain it back again. What happened was that the system (your lifestyle) exerted a force known as "homeostasis."

Homeostasis is the tendency of any system to resist change and to pull toward the status quo. If you make a change in one area, there will be a pull to resist that change and revert to what the system feels is normal. Sound familiar?

A diet takes a simplistic solution (eat less) and applies it to one part of the problem (food). This is what is described as a "first order change:" a band aid or quick fix that does not address things in a lasting way.

Mindful Life Weight Loss

This is precisely why we have the phenomenon of "yo-yo dieting." A first order change was what Laura was advised to do by a dietitian: Eat three meals, and stop binge eating at night. Clearly, such a solution is not adequate. And for most of us, our eating behavior might have other facets that require a more systemic solution.

Additionally, if we are not mindful of our habits and behaviors when we eat less, the power of homeostasis will increase calories (or reduce activity) as part of the system's effort to resist change. This will happen beneath the level of your awareness, as you subtly eat a little more here and there in response to your body's pull toward the status quo. This most frequently occurs when people increase their level of activity. Somehow, they manage to eat more calories to compensate. Mindfulness of this process is a big step in the direction of change.

Your metabolism also exerts its own pull toward homeostasis. While we are not going to delve into biology here, there is some validity to the idea that our bodies strive to remain at a certain set point weight. This doesn't mean you should give up! Rather, it means that you should simply factor this into your plan and be prepared. It may mean that your concept of ideal weight needs to be adjusted. Perhaps you can be healthy and happy at a heavier weight than you originally thought. Our concept of "ideal weight" is influenced by multiple factors: advertising, culture, and gender, to name a few. When we mindfully begin to separate what is healthy from what is trendy, fashionable, or culturally expected, we can arrive at a weight that is right for us, honoring our body's needs.

Mindful Life Weight Loss

The pull toward the status quo is a common occurrence in weight loss, and we should expect and prepare for it. This is especially true if change is too sudden or drastic, which is why you should aim for small, incremental changes.

An example of homeostasis happens frequently in couples when it comes to losing weight. A wife might want her spouse to lose weight. She may have been on his case for years and years. And when he finally does, what happens? She begins to unconsciously sabotage his weight loss. Maybe she throws a big party with his favorite foods. Maybe she starts to suddenly need him home when he is supposed to be working out...

Mindful Life in Action: Robert the Couch Potato turned Yogi's Homeostasis

Remember Robert from Chapter 2? He transformed his life in a major way by embracing a yoga lifestyle. While Robert was able to lose weight, reverse diabetes, and curb his alcohol consumption, he had a strong push back from other areas of his life. His wife, who was used to their old lifestyle and eating habits, continued to prepare unhealthy meals, bring home fast food, and indulge in nightly ice cream snacking. Robert frequently reported that his wife seemed to want to sabotage his success at every turn. Robert had to navigate his wife's ambivalent feelings about having a healthier husband, but also

Mindful Life Weight Loss

feeling like she was losing the old Robert. They sought couple's counseling to adjust to the changes. Robert learned that his new lifestyle was the beginning of another set of challenges to overcome.

Robert's wife did not try to "sabotage" him because she wanted to make his life miserable, and consciously undermine his weight loss. She acted the way she did because she was part of a system (the couple) and the system had been functioning a certain way for years. Suddenly, things changed and there was a natural tendency to restore it to the way it was.

Simply being aware of this tendency (mindfulness) can be very helpful in addressing it when it inevitably pops up. It can also take away some of the blame when we realize that we, and others, are not actively trying to sabotage anything. People behave in a predictable way because they are just doing what systems do.

Have you noticed this phenomenon in your weight loss journey? Have you lost weight, only to find that something popped up in your life to pull you back to your original weight---as if after all that paddling, the tide carried you right back to where you started? Write it down here:

Addressing a part of the issue with a simplistic solution is indeed like playing the game Whack-a-Mole. You hit one of the little mole heads only to have another pop up somewhere else. When you lack understanding of this process, you either frantically try to keep whacking moles, or give up. There is a better way: to use mindful awareness to figure out how the game works, and stay one step ahead.

How the Game Works: Relational Thinking

"How the game works" can be discovered by looking at the world through the lens of "relational thinking." Relational thinking is a key component of systems thinking. It always looks at the big picture and its interrelationships. It looks at the context of each behavior: when it happens, with whom, and where. It looks at patterns and similarities throughout your life. Relational thinking looks at all of the people in your life, and considers the part they play in the problem. It also spans generations and looks for patterns within families. Relational thinking looks for major life events, such as divorce, death, and job loss, and asks how those impact the problem. And finally, relational thinking understands that the solutions will involve friends, family, community, and many layers of a person's life. It is the essence of interconnectedness.

Everyone's situation is unique. The skill of mindful awareness will help you to notice the patterns, contexts, and relationships in your own life. Mindfulness will also help you to craft effective strategies, rather than simplistic "one size fits all" solutions.

.

Mindful Life Weight Loss

Effective Solutions

Another key concept of systems thinking is how we view problems and their solutions. Cause and effect are not necessarily closely related in time and space. This is why the simplistic statement "Just eat less!" doesn't work. It presumes the effect (being overweight) is closely related to its cause (amount of food). Systems thinking would certainly address food, but also inquire into other areas. The problem may really be the result of loneliness, stress, boredom, economic, or work issues. Our participants commonly report job stress and economic worries as a source of emotional eating. People working several jobs turn to junk food for quick energy. Looking at the larger picture, obesity is related to our troubled economy and low cost junk food, and thus its solution cannot be found without in some way addressing this larger context.

Take a moment to reflect on the cause and effect of your current struggles with weight. Can you think of other interrelationships that may be part of the cause? Write them down here:

There are multiple paths to the same goal. One person might lose weight by focusing on exercise and work/life balance. Another might rely more on diet and mindfulness. Either way, their end result will be weight loss in the context of a more Mindful Life. There is no

Mindful Life Weight Loss

one diet, magic pill, perfect exercise regimen. There is only a more Mindful Life, which is by its nature unique to the person. This program will help you find your individual path to your destination.

ACTION STEPS:

THIS WEEK, TAKE A LOOK AT THE TOPICS WE HAVE COVERED SO FAR:

MINDFULNESS

GOAL-SETTING

FOOD

MOVEMENT

EXERCISE

ARE THERE ANY PLACES WHERE YOU ARE FEELING STUCK?

ARE YOU SEEING ANY AREAS OF PUSH-BACK (THE TENDENCY TO MAINTAIN THE STATUS QUO)? ANY WHACK-A-MOLES? CONSIDER WHETHER THIS IS BECAUSE THE CHANGE WAS TOO SUDDEN, OR TOO DRASTIC. PERHAPS YOU CAN CONSIDER PULLING BACK.

ALSO REMEMBER YOUR VISION STATEMENT, AND GOALS ABOUT HABITS, FOOD, AND MOVEMENT. KEEP THEM POSTED IN PROMINENT PLACES. KEEP ENLISTING OTHER PEOPLE IN YOUR LIFE TO AID IN ACCOUNTABILITY AND SUPPORT.

9

Gaining Leverage, Increasing Momentum

USE ONE OUNCE TO DEFLECT 1,000 POUNDS
UNKNOWN ORIGIN – OFTEN USED SAYING IN TAI CHI CHUAN

Begin with three minutes of silence.

How did the week go?

What went well?

What areas of push-back from the system did you notice?

In this chapter, we will continue exploring systems thinking and learn how triggers, virtuous and vicious cycles, and leverage points impact our weight loss goals.

Habits consist of three elements (the habit trinity): trigger, actual behavior, and payoff. The trigger is whatever sets off the conditioned behavior. The English poet John Donne wrote, "No man is an island entire of itself; every man is a piece of the continent, a part of the main." When examining the triggers that cause us to engage in unhealthy behavior, we must look at the "continent" (the context) from which they arise.

We exist in the context of...

extended families (even if we don't speak to them!)
nuclear families
romantic relationships
co-workers
community
church, synagogue, community of faith
culture
gender
job
economic status
social status
race
and more

Which of these, or others, have the strongest pull in your life?

Mindful Life Weight Loss

Triggers

The habits that relate to our weight did not arise in a vacuum. They arose in contexts, and are maintained and supported by these contexts. Out of these contexts arise our triggers toward overeating. Knowledge of triggers is commonplace in the psychology of overeating (particularly emotional eating). Triggers are the first part of the "habit trinity."

A trigger is something in your external or internal environment that sparks behavior that is unhelpful to your weight loss goals. Think of Pavlov's dogs that salivated at the sound of the bell because they knew food (the reward) would soon follow. The bell was the trigger. Surprisingly, humans are not that different from Pavlov's dogs in that much of our behavior is automatic, triggered by a stimulus in our external or internal environment. This could be an event (an upsetting phone call, traffic jam, argument) or it could be an emotion (boredom, loneliness, anger). A trigger might even be a specific food, referred to as "trigger foods." Most often, it is a combination of internal and external factors that comprise a trigger.

Mindful Life in Action: Helen's Triggers

Like many Mindful Life participants, Helen struggled with emotional eating. For as long as she could remember, she had a sweet tooth and turned to sweets to soothe difficult emotions. Much of her diet was filled with healthy foods--fresh vegetables, lean meats, fruits, and whole grains. When she stuck to these foods, she had control over her eating behavior. She ate until she was full, did not overeat, and kept a stable weight. However, when Helen was under stress she reached for cookies and cakes for comfort. The stress was a trigger for her. But even worse, it triggered her to eat foods that, due to their chemical composition, trigger addictive eating behavior. Try as she may to limit herself to one or two cookies, she felt a total loss of control after eating sugary foods. "When I'm stressed and I reach for sweets, it's all over after the first bite" Helen declared after a particularly bad week. Helen came to understand that the sugar acted like a drug to her system when she was in certain vulnerable situations. Helen learned that her triggers were more complex than she originally thought: stress combined with the addictive qualities of certain foods created the context of her behavior.

Think of some triggers in your current life, and their context. List them here:

Examining triggers, and the context in which they arise, shines light on an important fact: we don't overeat simply because the food tastes good, or we "lack willpower" or "don't have discipline." We don't even always decide to overeat, as these behaviors are automatic, conditioned behaviors, rather than conscious decisions.

Mindful Life Weight Loss

Our behaviors that lead to weight gain are the result of habitual behaviors arising from multiple (often interrelated) contexts in our lives. Awareness of the trigger is half the battle, but too often people over-simplify triggers. For Helen, sugary foods were only a trigger in a particular context. At other times, Helen could have only one cookie. This is where systems thinking provides a vital relational, way of looking at the world. Awareness of the context of the trigger is crucial. The food itself is not solely the trigger--it is only part of it. The event itself is also only part of the trigger. Context is the trigger, and the context is unique to each of us.

Virtuous and Vicious Cycles

Perhaps you've been there. You are doing well on your weight loss plan. Then you are triggered to overeat. That leads to negative feelings--perhaps shame, disappointment, pessimism. In order to soothe the negative feelings, you eat some more. You notice your weight increasing. You feel miserable, dejected, and wonder "why bother." You quit going to the gym, and indulge further in unhealthy foods. And so on. This is a vicious cycle. In systems theory it is defined as a chain of events that reinforces itself through feedback loops. What I described above is a "feedback loop." One behavior (an "output") feeds back into the system as "input" and increases effects. Unless something interrupts this process, we all know where it will lead.

Mindfulness is the tool that interrupts the vicious cycle and helps transform it into a virtuous cycle. Group support (or individual coaching) is another tool, as the input from others can interrupt a vicious cycle.

A virtuous cycle occurs when positive behaviors produce positive effects that feed back into the system and produce more positive effects. In weight loss this happens when you begin to see good results from your new habits. Those good results produce positive feelings, which motivate you to persist in new habits, which result in weight loss. Mindfulness and group support are also key tools to maintaining the virtuous cycle in weight loss.

A small change that switches from a vicious cycle to a virtuous cycle is an example where a small effort can lead to big results, as one action stimulates an entire cycle.

Mindful Life in Action: Mike's Vicious Cycle Turns into a Virtuous Cycle

Mike was a middle-aged sales representative who came to us after trying to lose weight with a low carbohydrate weight loss program. Mike was from Italy and had many favorite foods that were culturally important to him. Many of these foods were carbohydrate-based foods. Mike's program required him to avoid many foods that he loved, and that made up part of his identity. Each week Mike would endure a lecture highlighting his areas of failure. And each week Mike would either not lose weight or gain a few pounds. He had a vicious cycle: a

Mindful Life Weight Loss

mismatched diet plan that he could not maintain, negative confrontations with his coach, feeling bad about himself for not losing weight, and then losing his motivation to keep trying. Fortunately, Mike interrupted this cycle when he had an epiphany: "I need to do this in a way that works for ME." This moment of mindfulness prompted him to join the Mindful Life program where he began a virtuous cycle. Highlighting his past successes, we helped him to expand upon his strengths, generate positive feelings, and in turn, lose weight. Mike loved to cook, so we helped him to adapt traditional recipes from his past to a healthier fare. Mike also loved to be a leader. We positioned Mike as a leader in some of the groups by having him talk about cooking and creating healthy recipes. Each week, Mike was able to feed into this virtuous cycle---even during plateaus---because he was learning how to capture and increase positive momentum. Mike turned a vicious cycle into a virtuous cycle with a moment of mindfulness.

Think of an example of a vicious cycle in your life:

Think of an example of a virtuous cycle in your life:

Payoffs as a Tool

When evaluating the habit cycle in the context of a system, it can be very helpful to start with the payoff. When you behave in a particular way, what are you really looking for? If you eat out of an uncontrollable desire for sugary foods, that says you are seeking happiness through physical sensation, comfort from pain, or perhaps stress relief.

Has it worked? If you gain too much weight, that leads to physical sensations that are quite uncomfortable---acid reflux, diabetes, high blood pressure. If the physical sensation of eating those foods did cause lasting happiness, then the more you ate the happier you would become. But that is not the case. The same goes for comfort and stress relief. Problems associated with obesity cause an increase in stress and painful feelings. You are not getting the payoff you are looking for.

Tracing the actions from the payoff side can give you an invaluable tool to question whether your current lifestyle is actually producing the benefits you originally imagined. You can use this as motivation to search for a better way to attain what you are looking for.

Leverage Points

Systems theory has provided us with another useful tool in weight loss: leverage points. Leverage is a concept that is borrowed from several fields and adapted to weight loss. For our purposes, leverage is the ability to effect change in a way that uses the minimal amount of effort to gain the maximum positive outcome.

Think of the many ways a person can go about losing weight (not all of them healthy):

going on a diet
taking diet pills

Mindful Life Weight Loss

surgery
hiring a chef
joining a gym
extreme exercise
going to a weight loss camp/clinic
adopting a restrictive diet
fasting
enforcing rules ("do and don't" behavior)
counseling
changing their mindset (cognitive-behavioral)
changing habits
setting goals
utilizing spirituality

Each of these areas represents a leverage point--a place in the system where you can effect change. However, not all leverage points are created equal. Systems theorist Donella Meadows states that there are twelve leverage points, and some are more influential--and less labor intensive--than others.

Each system—whether it is a corporation or an ecosystem---has its unique leverage points. In weight loss, leverage points are determined by what is practical, what is realistic, and what resonates with a person's lifestyle. Imagine a triangle. At the bottom of the triangle are physical interventions. They include everything from watching calories, increasing exercise, all the way to having surgery. These are very labor intensive. They require daily effort to sustain over a long period of time. Even surgery is far from a quick fix, as it requires lifelong monitoring of food intake and habits. If this sounds daunting, keep reading because you will learn how as you go up the triangle, you can achieve the same goals without as much hard work. The leverage points near the apex require the least effort for the greatest results.

The second tier includes behavioral interventions. These include setting goals, enrolling in structured programs, and working with rules and incentives. Included in this tier are programs designed by nutritionists, highly-structured short-term programs, and rewarding yourself for progress. Since this tier works at the level of behavior and creates an environment geared toward success, it requires less effort than the physical interventions. However, it usually relies on the help of structured programs or professionals. Strictly behavioral programs are best for targeted short-term results, or to jump start a longer-term process.

The third tier includes mental or psychological interventions. Motivation, confronting denial, entrenched habits, and larger lifestyle issues are part of this tier. This tier involves a shift in mindset. And finally, spirituality resides at the top. This tier comprises our highest personal values that may or may not correspond to a religion.

The two most influential leverage points are in the areas of shifting our mindset and in transcending our mindset (spirituality). These top tier leverage points have a way of infusing the lower tiers with energy and vitality. You will still implement physical and behavioral strategies, but they will be super-charged with meaningful, higher values. Without these higher values, physical and behavioral interventions are dry and uninspiring, and thus likely to fizzle out over the long term. When these higher values infuse your efforts, they allow you to achieve your goals in a way that feels effortless.

Mindful Life in Action: Steve Connects His Health Goals to His Spiritual Practice

From Steve Kanney, co-founder of Mindful Life Weight Loss: I was 26 years old. I was training in martial arts, working hard at my job, and taking care of my father who had Alzheimer's disease. My mother had already passed away. My father's life rested upon my shoulders. But the stress was too much for me to handle. I remember sitting in a doctor's office listening to him tell me I had cancer. He thought I probably only had a few months. I was 26 years old, barely knowing what life was about, and I was about to lose it. Aside from the shock, I was awash in a sea of pain. I had this life, I never tried to figure out what it was really for, and I squandered it. I knew I wanted to live, and I knew I wanted to make my life meaningful. That meant taking care of myself so I could take care of my father, at least first. The surgery turned out much better than expected, but I was told I may need medication for high cholesterol. At age 26! My diet was terrible. I wanted to live, so I read this book called The 8-Week Cholesterol Cure. Sure enough, in 8 weeks my cholesterol dropped by over 20% and has even declined further over the next 25 years (It normally goes up with age). That was it. Knowing that I was going to live gave me the motivation to stay healthy so I could live

Mindful Life Weight Loss

the rest of my life with meaning and spiritual purpose. These top tier leverage points make it easy to have the motivation I need to make healthy choices.

Mindfulness helps us to address weight loss from the two most powerful leverage points, while also encompassing all the other leverage points as needed. Like Steve, you can find a way to connect your spiritual values with your health goals, thus making your efforts feel effortless.

Take a moment to consider some of your top tier leverage points. What is most meaningful to you? What are your highest personal and/or spiritual values? How can you link them to your weight loss goals? List them here:

Knowledge of triggers, cycles, and leverage points will help you intentionally create positive momentum in your weight loss journey.

Action Steps:

Exercise:

Take one scenario from your life and identify the trigger.

One common trigger is:

Mindful Life Weight Loss

The context of this trigger is (when does it happen, with whom, where, at what times of the year, i.e. holidays, seasons, etc.):

Now, brainstorm a strategy to address this trigger. Factor in what you have just learned about leverage points. Remember, you are halfway there because you have become mindful of the problem.

One strategy is:

Put this strategy for addressing triggers to work in your life this week! Record your experience below.

If you are having trouble with your motivation, why don't you see what you are really motivated to do? What is the payoff for the actions you spend the most time/effort in doing? What is the ultimate objective? Is it working or is it self-defeating? Is there a better way?

Also recall your Vision Statement, and goals surrounding habits, food, and movement.

Continue to investigate what kind of exercise you might like to explore.

Mindful Life Weight Loss

10

Green Time vs. Screen Time

> WHEN ONE TUGS AT A SINGLE THING IN NATURE, HE FINDS THAT IT IS ATTACHED TO THE REST OF THE WORLD.
> JOHN MUIR

Begin with three minutes of silence.

What went well this week?

Have you identified your most powerful leverage points?

Which areas need improvement?

By this point, you have walked down a path of weight loss that truly includes your whole life: from food and movement to how to be mindful of your life and use your life's interconnectedness to your advantage. However, there is one area that we have not addressed: nature.

Don't worry, we are not talking about going on a wilderness adventure, or hiking the Appalachian Trail. We are talking about what exists footsteps from your front door, just outside your office window. What you drive through on your way to work. What you walk through as you get out of your car and walk into the store. Nature, or "green time." Anything that is outside---even if you live and work in an urban environment---is "nature."

We live in a world where people are spending increasing amounts of time indoors. Consider some of the following examples, and reflect on how they may contribute to the obesity epidemic:

- People spend less time outdoors now than at any point in human history.
- Recess for children is getting shorter, and in some cases eliminated.
- Some people (both adults and children) spend their entire days sitting in a chair under unnatural lighting.
- Sleep disturbances are rampant.
- We spend an unprecedented amount of time staring at a screen---our laptops, televisions, phones, Kindle readers, video games or workstations.
- Our natural sleep rhythm is disrupted by exposure to artificial light, particularly looking at a screen right up until the time we sleep.
- There is an app for everything.

- For some people, the only time they spend outdoors involves walking from their car to another indoor space.
- We drive everywhere, as our towns and cities are not pedestrian-friendly and in some cases unsafe due to drugs and violence.
- Unstructured outdoor play has been replaced with supervised indoor playtime, due to fears about safety.

Consider your life now, as it is. How much time do you spend outdoors? What factors keep you indoors? Which of the insights above resonates most with you?

There is a clear link, as the more time you spend in front of a screen (especially TV) the higher your BMI is likely to be. You can probably already see how your screen time impacts your weight. But it may have a bigger impact than you think.

Counteract your excessive indoor and "screen time" and see how increasing your exposure to nature can affect your weight in five key ways. When you take a few steps outside of your door, you are taking more steps on the path to a Mindful Life.

Mindful Life in Action: Walking My Daughter to School

A few years ago, one of my goals was to walk more. I felt that I was spending too much time indoors and wanted to make a change. Yet, there were always work demands and household responsibilities keeping me from getting outside and enjoying a walk in nature. So, I set a small measurable goal. I would walk my daughter home from school every day. I linked my goal of "walking more" to something I already did: walking my daughter home from school. The school was about 1/2 to 3/4 mile away. I couldn't walk her to school because I needed to drive somewhere directly after dropping her off. Yet walking her home was easy. That amounted to an extra 90+ miles walked per year. 90 miles! For an activity that took about 15 minutes round-trip every day. I discovered that it actually took me less time to walk than drive since I got caught in horrible after-school traffic. This small change rippled outward as my daughter and I spent quality time together, enjoyed the seasons (the good and the bad), reduced stress from being in traffic, and got to know others in our neighborhood.

Spending more time in nature, and less time in front of a screen, helps to:

1. *Decrease sedentary time.* Screen-based activities increase sedentary time. Any activity that is done in front of a screen is often done from a seated position. Before you know it, you realize that you have been sitting looking at a screen all day and all evening. How does that make you feel physically? Mentally? Probably not good. Often, at the end of a stressful, sedentary day, the only physical release people can get is to eat sugary or fat-laden snacks that-- in the short-term--boost feel-good chemicals. Unfortunately, they also boost your weight.

Mindful Life Weight Loss

Most activities done outdoors involve movement: walking the kids to school, errands, biking, raking, gardening, outdoor chores, hiking, walking the dog, etc.

2. *Decrease levels of stress.* The research is clear. When you spend time in a natural environment (suburban yards and urban parks included) your body responds by lowering blood pressure and reducing cortisol (stress hormone). Additionally, there is increased activity in the part of our nervous system responsible for calm (the parasympathetic nervous system). This benefit can also be derived from indoor plants or by looking out the window at a beautiful natural scene. Additional research on the health benefits of time in nature can be found in *Your Brain on Nature* by Eva M. Selhub, MD and Alan C. Logan, ND.

Stress is one of the key causes of overeating, so anything that decreases stress in a healthy way is an excellent way to combat stress-related eating. The calming sensation that you get from comforting foods can also be obtained from time spent in nature.

3. *Put you in touch with community.* Sadly, in some communities, people do not even know their neighbors. Loneliness and isolation are "sleeper" causes of obesity. They are contributing factors that often do not make it onto people's radar when they assess their weight struggles. Getting outside more, even if it is just to go for a daily 15 minute walk around your neighborhood, means you might connect

more with those around you. I noticed this when I walked my daughter home from school. I felt a greater connection to my neighbors, the natural world, and my community from this short walk.

Who knows what the ripple effect of this will be. I remember in my own life back in the early '00s, I started a daily walk (alone). One neighbor saw me from her window and joined me. Then another, and another. Soon there were five of us. Several of us had small children so we strapped them into the stroller and we all walked five days a week. We bonded as new mothers. One of us brought a dog. I made new friends, and my brief walk turned into a much longer walk (sometimes nearly 2 hours) because we all enjoyed the social opportunity. This was a true ripple effect.

4. *Create a calm, focused mental state.* Screen time requires a certain set of mental skills---those of "directed attention" or "voluntary attention." This is the sustained effort you need to do your work obligations, read emails, answer texts, and all of the various ways we spend our "screen time." This type of attention requires a lot of energy, and over time causes mental fatigue. One has to resist the continual pull of distracting thoughts to maintain focus.

Contrast this to "involuntary attention" which is when you are doing something more free-form; walking, jogging, daydreaming, gardening, or being effortlessly absorbed in a task (the "flow" state).

Mindful Life Weight Loss

Studies have been done to see if we can combat our cognitive fatigue by spending some time in natural settings. The results were that we can. Spending time outdoors, in natural light, fresh air, amidst natural sounds, is like pressing the reset button on our nervous system.

The more you can bring brief periods of this state into your life, the more mindful your life can become. This mindfulness can then extend to mindfulness of your habits, and eating behaviors.

5. *Help you to develop a more holistic view of yourself in the ecosystem.* As you become more mindful, you begin to see things beyond just yourself. Just as you are not simply your weight, and your weight is not only about food. This journey toward a Mindful Life is not simply about you. It is about our families, our communities, and the whole planet.

That apple that you ate may have come from Chile. In that one bite, you are connected with a farmer in another continent. Your choices affect him and his family. A drought or disaster in one area affects us in America.

When we spend most of our time indoors, watching nature on a screen and rarely feeling the sun on our faces, it is easy to forget that we are all connected in a real way. This isn't just a platitude. The more time we spend away from screens and out in the actual world, the more real this will become for us.

Mindful Life in Action: Josh's "All You Can Eat" Vacation

Mindful Life Weight Loss

Josh had been in the Mindful Life program for four months and had lost 15 pounds. He and his wife were scheduled to go on an all-inclusive vacation with constant access to food. Josh felt that in order to enjoy his vacation, he needed to partake in rich, indulgent foods in large quantities. Josh crafted a plan that allowed for him to enjoy the foods he loved in moderation. However, he could not shake the idea that vacation equalled unrestricted eating. On the other hand, Josh did not want to gain back the weight he lost. We asked him to shine the light of mindfulness on the theme of "rewards" and "enjoyment" in life. He thought about what he enjoyed and why, and the many non-food ways he could "feed" himself on vacation. Josh concluded that he would limit his food indulgences to three meals a day (of whatever foods/amounts he wanted), and abstain from snacking. During the rest of his time he would feed himself with tropical sunshine, swimming, shimmering water, natural beauty, naps on a hammock, hikes, and fresh air. Josh discovered that nature fed him. It fed his senses, his soul, and his body in a profound way. It calmed his mind, and gave him a sense of awe far beyond the buffet at the resort. Josh was able to have his "all you can eat" vacation, but natural beauty was his food.

How I Created the "Green for 15" Challenge

When I was a graduate student studying Marriage and Family Therapy, I took a class in Community Psychology. My final project was to design a simple, low cost, grass roots intervention that could address a community mental health problem. I chose the issue

Mindful Life Weight Loss

of stress and decided to create a way for people to spend more time outdoors. I called it the Green for 15 challenge. The idea behind Green for 15 was to create a challenge where people would commit to 15 minutes each day---not necessarily all at one time---spent mindfully outdoors. This goal was small enough to be attainable by just about anyone, yet had big "ripple effect" potential. I started with myself and my family and had excellent results. My professor took the challenge as well. I made the Green for 15 challenge an integral part of the Mindful Life Weight Loss program and am continually inspired at how a small amount of time outdoors can have big results.

Green for 15 Challenge

Try taking the Green for 15 challenge. It is simple: commit to spending 15 minutes a day outside. It doesn't even have to be all at once.

Walk an extra block to get coffee.
Get off one bus stop earlier and walk the difference.
Go for a walk after dinner for a few minutes.
Park farther away.

Fifteen minutes isn't really that much time, but you may see a ripple effect that is really positive. Remember my walking adventure where I added 90 miles in one year and barely noticed. That time encouraged me to make several other small changes: I walked my dog more, spent more time outdoors as a result of buying warmer winter clothing, did more yard work, and walked other places.

Remember, small changes make big results!

Mindful Life Weight Loss

List 3 ways you can add a few minutes of outdoor time in your life:

1.

2.

3.

ACTION STEP:

COMMIT TO THE GREEN FOR 15 CHALLENGE THIS WEEK. ADD IT TO YOUR VISION STATEMENT. REMEMBER TO KEEP YOUR VISION STATEMENT IN A PROMINENT PLACE!

11

Beyond Ourselves

> AT ANY MOMENT YOU HAVE A CHOICE THAT EITHER LEADS YOU CLOSER TO YOUR SPIRIT OR FURTHER AWAY FROM IT.
> THICH NHAT HANH

Begin with three minutes of silence.

How did the week go?

What went well? What else? And what else?

How did the Green for 15 challenge work out?

What were some ways that you worked outdoor time into your life? What were some obstacles to this challenge?

How has the exploration of exercise been going?

What have you discovered?

Mindful Life Weight Loss

This week we will be discussing how to put it all together, and what this means for our world. We've covered a lot ground quickly, and juggling it all at once likely still feels overwhelming. That's okay; we're still in the process of learning. Rely on mindfulness to lead you, and commit yourself to avoiding the self-judgment that will impede your journey.

To do this, consider your higher purpose for your weight loss. People are often motivated to lose weight because of the effect it has on their loved ones. Many people are concerned that they will die from obesity-related conditions, and the effect that will have on their families. Others are limited by their health problems, and feel they cannot do everything they want to do in life. These are excellent motivations for losing weight, because they expand the issue outside the realm of simply "weight loss."

Losing weight for its own sake can feel like an uphill battle, but when you tap into your deeper motivations, you gain momentum. What is your burning desire? What gets you up out of bed every morning? What makes you feel alive, meaningful, and significant? What makes you, you?

Use your mindfulness practice to reach down to your core self. It is here that you can get in touch with your deepest values and link those to your health goals. There is no other way to make your new lifestyle work long term. One of the reasons why diets don't work is that they lack a profound underlying motivation. Motivation needs fuel. Think of it as a fire that needs to be continually fed so that it does not die out. Looking good in a bathing suit, achieving a BMI, or a "pounds lost" goal are simply not powerful enough to underscore a complete lifestyle shift. They lack passion, and are thus subject to being displaced by more compelling habits. During weak moments, you need something even more enjoyable than chocolate cake, or that provides even more peace than the comfort of a binge eating episode.

These values don't have to be spiritual, but they often are. Service to others, love for family, devotion to God, making a difference in the world are all "spiritual" values that people have linked to their health goals.

Mindful Life in Action: Alicia Got Healthy for the Animals

Alicia was a devoted animal lover. She rescued animals from the streets, rehabilitated them, and found homes for them. She also had a lovely menagerie of animals in her home. She realized that she needed to be as healthy as possible, and live as long as she could, to care for her animals, and to rescue other animals. She felt that this was her life's mission, as her animal companions were what lifted her out of a deep depression many years prior. Alicia had many areas of her life that were troublesome besides her weight. She also struggled with conflictual relationships. However, Alicia was able to keep her love for animals as her motivation and found the energy she needed to take small step after small step. Her homework was to go home each night, and when she looked into the eyes of her animal companions say "This is the reason why I stay on track."

Other core values may have to do with your identity. Who are you, really? Some people discover a new identity as an athlete, yogi, martial artist, or runner. They embody those identities through their weight loss journey. Then, after they have lost the weight, the attributes of their new identities are habits that come naturally to them. Robert became a dedicated yoga practitioner. He adopted a whole foods yogic diet, and that became who he was. He was able to switch his identity from a sedentary person who ate a lot of processed food, to an active yogi who aspired to a certain lifestyle.

And still other core values may relate to a life passion or goal. Recall Laura who used to binge eat and stay up late at night. When we discussed what she would do with her time if she was up all day, she said she would go to a cafe and work on writing her life story. This was her gift to the world, and spending the day sleeping was preventing her from doing this work. This deep goal fueled her motivation to perform the very hard work of regulating her sleeping and eating schedule.

Think about what motivates you? What lights your fire? Link this to your health goals and you will super-charge your efforts.

Reaping the Benefits of a Mindful Life

Mindful Life Weight Loss

As you make your way along the path of a Mindful Life, delving deeper and deeper into your core motivations, you see that when you become more mindful your life opens up. You don't just lose weight. You gain health and vitality.

You also gain expanded awareness. What does this awareness mean for you? Here are five ways that living a mindful life can benefit your personal life as well as the lives of those around you.

1. *Mindful living helps to slow things down.* When mindfulness is introduced into your life, behaviors are no longer automatic, knee-jerk reactions. The mindfulness muscle helps you to pause.

Rather than eating vast amounts of food without even realizing it, or making food choices at the supermarket based on conditioned factors, the mindful pause puts space between the impulse and the action. In the space of the few seconds you take a few breaths, tune in to your body, and become aware, you find that you make different choices. Having this space between the impulse and the action is the bedrock of habit change, as well as the beginning of more intentional living.

Sometimes the difference between whether you eat the entire quart of ice cream, or go out for a walk, is as little as 10 deep breaths. Sometimes all it takes is to slow things down so you can hear your own inner wisdom, and the wisdom of your body. This is not about living life in slow motion, but bringing things back to a normal pace.

Our modern world comes at us at lightning speed, but a mindful life feels slower and more manageable. For a large part of our history, we had natural, built-in pauses. We had to grow, prepare, hunt, or cook our food. We had to work countless hours to earn money to buy luxuries (pre-credit card days). We had to wait for the mail to arrive, or travel to see someone face to face.

Today, everything happens in an instant, including our choices about food and lifestyle. Mindfulness introduces a natural pause that temporarily takes you off of the insane treadmill, and puts you in touch with your best interests.

2. *Mindful living helps you to see things more clearly.* We have begun each chapter with a few minutes of mindfulness. This has been the "workout" that has strengthened the mindfulness muscle, like lifting barbells or doing push-ups. When this muscle gets stronger and becomes a way of life, you will notice that you can see everything more clearly---your thoughts, emotions, motivations, and behaviors. You may even find that you experience your body differently, getting a clearer picture of when you are full, what kinds of food your body needs, and how certain foods make you feel.

Mindful living is really about getting to know your own mind. Imagine your mind is like one of those snow globes. The busyness of everyday life is like having the globe constantly shaken. The liquid never has a chance to be undisturbed, and thus is continually clouded with "snow." When you begin living mindfully, you stop the constant shaking and jostling. The debris settles, and you experience an increase in clarity.

Of course, this doesn't happen immediately. Quite often, people first begin to notice how cluttered and chaotic their mind is. They are noticing the white flecks of snow swirling around--something they simply thought was normal. However, with time and practice, that will begin to settle, and the new normal will be an increased sense of clarity.

3. *Mindful living helps you to live with greater intention.* Once you begin to slow down and take notice, you can direct your life according to your intentions. You become an actor, not a reactor.

This is simply not possible when you are being shaken, jostled, and pulled in all directions. Your focus improves. New habits develop that are in line with your values. It no longer becomes a struggle to be more active, or to eat healthy foods because it is your clear, undivided intention to do so.

Living with intention is only possible when you are able to unite body-mind-spirit. When the body is doing one thing (surfing the web while eating chips and drinking soda), the mind is distracted and cluttered, and the spirit is a tiny voice drowned out by the chatter, your intentions are merely "nice ideas" that never come to fruition.

Living mindfully, you unite all parts of yourself and really begin to live the life you have always wanted to live. The average person whittles away several hours on the internet doing nothing in particular. Imagine what could be accomplished if that time was aligned with their intentions? Mindfulness inspires us to ask such questions.

4. *Mindful living helps you to see connections.* Everything really is connected. With globalization, now more than ever. Our choices affect everyone and everything around us. Your lifestyle is not just yours, it is the planet's. A small percentage of the global population is responsible for most of the resources. Thich Nhat Hanh refers to this as Mindful Consumption and details it in his book *Savor*.

Americans decide they like beef and miles of rain forest are destroyed for cattle grazing. Cheap clothing means child labor in Indonesia. Plastic and disposable everything means the oceans are clogged with waste. Over-reliance on antibiotics and pharmaceuticals means that our waterways are awash in drugs excreted and flushed down the toilets. I recently learned that much of the wild-caught shrimp comes from enslaved humans on fishing boats in Asia. I had no idea. Our most personal daily choices affect everyone around us.

The typical reaction to such information is to have "suffering overload," tune out, and continue on with life as usual. What can we really do but throw up our hands in powerlessness and despair? Mindful living is the middle ground--the realistic answer. Mindful living is being aware of the effect of the connection between our behavior and the planet, and not tuning out in despair.

Mindful Life Weight Loss

We do what we can do in our own small lives, in our own unique ways. Can we do everything? No. Can we do something? Yes. And each one of us can decide, using mindful awareness, what that something is.

I remember listening to an introduction for a very accomplished author. He was in his seventies, and had a staggeringly impressive list of accolades. When the announcer was finished with the long list of awards and publications, the audience was silent with awe. The author simply waved his hand and said "I did a couple things a year. I'm an old man. It adds up."

That is how it is when you expand your awareness of the connections between your actions and the planet. You can't do everything. But you choose what you can realistically do, do a few things (think small and attainable), and over time it will add up to something significant.

5. *Mindful living will increase your sense of compassion.* A natural result of mindfulness is increased compassion. Most people take pleasure in helping others. When mindful awareness is increased, one of the first things to go is self-judgment. Recall, that our definition of mindfulness is non-judgmental awareness. Shame, guilt, low self-esteem, and self-hate are frequent issues for people struggling with weight. With mindful awareness, you learn how to be compassionate toward yourself. Naturally, that will expand outward to others. It is impossible to embody true compassion for others without having it for yourself first. Prioritizing your own self-care leads to a greater capacity to care for others. This is one of the

key elements to living a Mindful Life, and indeed, a key component of a happy life.

Think about one area of your life that you might like to begin to make a change that impacts the planet. Set a small and attainable goal here, and then re-write on your Vision Statement:

I will:

ACTION STEPS:

ACHIEVE YOUR SMALL, ATTAINABLE, AND ACCOUNTABLE GOAL WITH REGARD TO MAKING THE WORLD A BETTER PLACE.

BRAINSTORM HOW YOU CAN MAKE YOURSELF ACCOUNTABLE FOR THIS GOAL:

I WILL BE ACCOUNTABLE FOR THIS GOAL IN THE FOLLOWING WAY:

I WILL SET MY ENVIRONMENT UP FOR SUCCESS IN THE FOLLOWING WAY:

Mindful Life Weight Loss

Achieve this goal this week!

You have begun--and gained momentum in-- several important areas:
One habit change
A food-related goal
A movement goal
Exploring exercise
Green for 15
And now, a goal for the planet.

Remember to add to your Vision Statement and keep it posted in prominent places.

Mindful Life Weight Loss

12

Emotional Eating

> BREATHING IN, I CALM BODY AND MIND. BREATHING OUT, I SMILE. DWELLING IN THE PRESENT MOMENT I KNOW THIS IS THE ONLY MOMENT.
> THICH NHAT HANH

Emotional Eating: The Basics

In modern life, the easy availability of delicious food has resulted in food being used as a way of coping with difficult emotions. We eat in response to our feelings, rather than in response to a true sensation of hunger.

But we don't need a formal definition to know what emotional eating is. Most of us are familiar with emotional eating. "Comfort foods" earned their name because of their ability to soothe negative emotions.

Much of our eating behavior can be classified as "emotional." Now this isn't necessarily a bad thing, since emotions fuel so much of our behavior. We humans are emotional creatures (far more emotional than we care to admit). It only becomes problematic when it is automatic, and when we get swept away on the "express train" from negative emotion---> food without any other choices along the way. Mindfulness interrupts this "express train" and re-routes it to a variety of positive coping behaviors.

Emotional Regulation

All emotions need to be regulated in some way. When we regulate our emotions, we make them more manageable, more tolerable, and reduce the likelihood of reacting on impulse and doing something we regret later (like finishing the whole gallon of ice cream). Emotional eating is one way that we attempt to regulate our emotions. However, since it brings with it so many additional problems, it is not a particularly useful way.

During an emotional eating episode, we experience a temporary sense of comfort as our energy is shifted away from the distressing emotion and toward digestion. People typically consume high fat, high carbohydrate foods which prompt the release of serotonin (a neurotransmitter that calms and soothes). Emotional eating is a quick fix in that it distracts from the emotion and creates a physical sense of calm.

The temporary calm (we'll call it "false calm") of emotional eating is in fact the calm before the storm. After the calm wears off, emotional eating episodes trigger feelings of shame, hopelessness, and various other negative emotions.

Mindful Life Weight Loss

Emotional eating can also be a prelude to "all or nothing thinking," a common cognitive distortion that makes people lose momentum on their weight loss program: since I wasn't 100 percent perfect, I might as well abandon healthy eating altogether. "All or nothing thinking" sets off a vicious cycle.

Mindfulness: How it Can Help Interrupt the Cycle

Taking a few mindful breaths is like hitting a pause button. It helps you to take a step back and slow down, and redirect to other coping behaviors. Emotional eating tends to happen automatically. We may be aware that there is some distressing emotion triggering overeating. However, like an express train, it rapidly leaves the station before we can really investigate our experience. Before we know it, we are engaging in unhealthy eating behaviors. Mindfulness helps us to actually identify and understand what is going on.

However, mindfulness is more than raw awareness. Mindfulness is compassionate awareness. So, when we become aware that we are eating because of hurt, stress, or anger, self-compassion can soothe those emotions right away like a mother soothes her crying child

Think of our emotions as a crying infant, and we are its mother. Mindfulness occurs when the mother holds the crying infant, staying present with it, and giving it loving attention. Emotional eating, on the other hand, is like the mother putting food into the infant's mouth every time it cries. If she did this, she would never be able to discern the infant's real needs, or tell if the infant was truly hungry.

As we have learned, mindfulness helps us to become more comfortable with discomfort, and we are better able to tolerate distressing emotions. Getting comfortable with discomfort via safe and non-threatening activities, such as yoga, meditation, or martial arts training, is an excellent way to help deal with emotional eating. Next time a distressing emotion arises, the "mindfulness muscle" has already been developed, and we will be less likely to soothe with food.

Mindfulness gives us choices. Our emotional eating express train is interrupted by a stop at "Mindfulness." From there, the train is free to travel to an endless number of other positive coping behaviors. Rather than an automatic destination of "eating," we can now choose from any number of positive, healthy coping behaviors. This is how a vicious cycle is transformed into a virtuous cycle, as positive coping behaviors lead to positive feelings, which lead to more positive behaviors.

Mindful Life in Action: Amy's Different Choices

Amy was a participant in our program working through her issues with emotional eating. She had learned that one of her triggers was conflictual situations at her job. Whenever she would have a bad day at work, she would come home and binge on high-carbohydrate foods as a way of dealing with the stress. As Amy progressed through our program and honed her skill of mindfulness, she was better able to interrupt her habitual behavior and engage in healthier coping behaviors. One night, Amy came home from a bad day at work and felt the familiar urge to self-soothe through eating. But instead, she did a guided meditation practice that she had on an app. After, she pulled a book off of the shelf. It was a self-help book that had been recommended to her. She made a cup of tea and read a chapter in the book that was particularly relevant to her job situation. She then went for a walk to sort out her feelings about her day at work. She did not overeat that night. Mindfulness gave her a brief pause. In that pause she was able to make a different choice. Amy was able to find that pause because she had been practicing for several months.

Notice how Amy had improved clarity about what she really needed. Amy had become better at tolerating distressing emotions, so there was more spaciousness in her decision-making process. Amy had now opened up more choices as to how she could properly tend to these emotions.

All of these healthier coping behaviors were available to Amy because she interrupted the emotional eating express train with mindfulness. When Amy chooses one of these behaviors, she will also experience positive emotions (i.e. feel good about herself, increase her confidence, gain a sense of momentum), rather than feel the shame and guilt that follow an emotional eating episode. Amy can now initiate a virtuous cycle.

The Brain on Mindfulness

So, what happens to the brain when we take a mindful pause by taking a few mindful breaths? Mindfulness practice activates the part of our brain responsible for decision-making (the prefrontal cortex) rather than raw emotion. This part of our brain helps us to make decisions---especially decisions that are in line with our goals (as opposed to impulsive behaviors that derail our goals).

Don't Wait Until You Have a Problem to Practice

You should begin a mindfulness practice at times when you are not feeling distressed and practice it regularly at times when you are not feeling distressed.

Many people learn a new mindfulness skill, such as the mindful breathing practice. They practice it only once or twice, and wait until they are in a highly distressing situation to try it out. Then, they apply their newly-minted mindfulness skill and are discouraged that it didn't work. Then, sadly, they may give up on the practice.

It didn't work because it is a new skill. It is unrealistic to expect to perform any new skill under duress. It is far better to practice the new skill when we are not under stress, or when we are only mildly stressed, to build up the "mindfulness muscle." Then, when it is needed it will be strong and capable.

Mindful Life Weight Loss

Additionally, a regular mindfulness practice helps us to reset our triggers altogether. Over time, as our general level of stress decreases, our triggers reset accordingly. What used to be an "8" on the distress scale is now down to a "5." With regular practice, we can raise our overall sense of well-being.

13

Measuring Success

Congratulations! You have come a long way on your path to sustainable weight loss.

You also may have taken a few steps back, and encountered a few obstacles along the way. Your motivation may have started high and then faltered a few times. You also may have walked away from the path, only to return. Know that this is completely normal. Setbacks are a natural part of change. They are to be expected, and factored into the plan. As you conclude this program and continue on your path, it is important to understand two things: 1) how you can gauge your own success when you step out on your own; and 2) how you can sustain your success while dealing with natural setbacks and fluctuating motivation.

How to Gauge Success

Being able to gauge success accurately is a very important skill. Many people become discouraged and lose motivation simply because they are inaccurately gauging their own success. They only see one narrow metric, and perceive themselves as "failing." They don't recognize important gains in other areas.

Each chapter asked the question: "what went well?" This question trains your mind to highlight areas of competency. Going forward, you will need to adopt a similar way of gauging your success--one that factors in areas of competency as well as areas of need.

Prior to beginning this program, the scale (or the mirror) may have been your only metric of success. I know from personal experience that linking your success to the number on a scale is a merciless taskmaster, as well as a surefire killer of joy. There is a better way. Use the skill of mindfulness to create your own holistic rubric of success.

You decide which factors are important, and make a custom-made rubric. A rubric is a standard of performance with clearly stated expectations. For many, their only rubric is "pounds lost" or whether they fit in a pair of jeans. After you have completed this program, you should have many other metrics with which to measure success. These metrics will encompass the totality of your experience, rather than just a sliver.

Mindful Life Rubric: How Am I Doing?

I have established a regular mindfulness practice _____ times per week.

I have made self-care a priority.   5 4 3 2 1

I am practicing self-compassion.   5 4 3 2 1

More of my food choices are whole, unprocessed foods.   5 4 3 2 1

I feel more energetic.   5 4 3 2 1

I have increased my daily level of activity.   5 4 3 2 1

I am participating in an enjoyable form of exercise _____ times per week.

My health outcomes have improved (A1C, blood pressure, etc.).   5 4 3 2 1

I am spending more time in nature.   5 4 3 2 1

I am spending less time in front of the screen.   5 4 3 2 1

I have lost _____ pounds and am _____ pounds from my goal weight.

I am managing my stress.   5 4 3 2 1

Mindful Life Weight Loss

I am coping with emotional eating through positive coping behaviors.	5 4 3 2 1
I am thinking beyond myself, living to benefit those around me.	5 4 3 2 1
I feel happier.	5 4 3 2 1
I am gaining insight into my behaviors.	5 4 3 2 1
I am connecting with others for support and encouragement.	5 4 3 2 1
I am getting a good night of sleep.	5 4 3 2 1
I am tracking my daily food with a food diary or app (myfitnesspal, etc.)	5 4 3 2 1

What we measure, we are more likely to achieve. Above is an example of a measurement rubric that can be adjusted to your own personal vision of success (5 is the highest). Use all of them, a few of them, or create your very own right here:

Mindful Life Weight Loss

What are your key indicators of success?

When scoring, keep this in mind: If you are scoring high in only one area of this list, that is still a valuable indicator of success.

Mindful Life in Action: Anna Puts Herself First

Anna was a 35 year old marketing manager who shared a house with her parents. She often found herself helping her parents with miscellaneous tasks around the house, running their errands, and even accompanying them to social events. As a result of her parents' demands, Anna had trouble maintaining her weight loss routines, such as making it to the group class, and going to the gym. For the first several weeks of our program, Anna lost very little weight. Instead, Anna's goals were to improve her boundaries with her parents so that she could put her health first. It took some time for Anna to open a discussion about her own needs, and how important it was for her to say no to many of her parents' requests. If Anna was only looking at the number on the scale, she would have been discouraged by her progress. However, we helped Anna to see that she was laying the groundwork for future success, and that was a valuable foundation. This knowledge helped to keep Anna's motivation high, as well to include her parents in her weight loss goals as supporters rather than saboteurs.

Mindful Life Weight Loss

With firmer boundaries in place, Anna was able to enroll in a fun fitness class, and better meet her own needs.

This is a lifestyle, not a diet. If you have not lost any weight one week-- or even if you have gained weight-- but you have made significant strides in practicing self-care like Anna, that is a win. If you have had a bad week (or month),don't despair. Don't use lower scores as opportunities to beat yourself up, but rather as part of a feedback loop to course correct.

If you have learned something about yourself, that is success: ("I am gaining insight into my behaviors...") Customize your rubric to provide yourself with useful data that both reflects your successes, self-knowledge, and areas in need of improvement.

Conclusion

Take a moment and reflect upon how far you have come. Know that the decision to improve your health will have a ripple effect through your own world, and the world in general. Your positive changes will influence your children and those around you. Perhaps you have already seen the fruits of your practice.

This is only the beginning. The skills you have learned in this book will help you to expand upon your efforts. Now that you know how to set and achieve small goals, you can move onto incrementally bigger goals. And as long as you continue to practice mindfulness and cover the five areas of weight loss, you are on the path to success. You can continue to revise and use your Vision Statement and Mindful Life rubric. You are set up to lose weight, and to maintain a healthy weight, in a way that is natural and enjoyable. Because you have activated and developed the skill of mindfulness, you can use that awareness as your guide. The days of miserable diets are over. You can finally make peace with your weight.

Best wishes on this exciting journey. May you have good health and happiness!

Mindful Life Weight Loss

Never Give Up

No matter what is going on
Never give up
Too much energy in your country is spent
developing the mind
Instead of the heart
Develop the heart
Be compassionate
Not just to your friends, but to everyone
Be compassionate
Work for peace in your heart and in the world
Work for peace
And I say it again
Never give up
No matter what is happening
No matter what is going on around you
Never give up

His Holiness the XIVth Dalai Lama

Mindful Life Weight Loss

Additional Resources

Mindfulness

Savor: Mindful Eating, Mindful Life

Thich Nhat Hanh, Lilian Cheung

Excellent foundation in mindful eating and living. Written by a Zen Master and a doctor of nutrition, this book provides a scientific and a spiritual foundation.

How to Eat (Mindful Essentials)

Thich Nhat Hanh

This book contains short meditations that will transform how you eat every day.

Mindful Eating: A Guide to Rediscovering a Healthy and Joyful Relationship with Food (Includes CD)

Jan Chozen Bays, MD

A Zen priest and MD offers very practical and insightful tools to transform your relationship with food.

Mindful Life Weight Loss

Eat Q: Unlock the Weight-Loss Power of Emotional Intelligence

Susan Albers, PsyD

In-depth tools for emotional eating. Psychologist Susan Albers brings the tools of behavioral science to explore emotions and eating in the context of mindfulness.

Mindless Eating: Why We Eat More Than We Think

Brian Wansink

A research psychologist turns the studies of the restaurant industry around to help us gain control of the 200+ daily decisions we make about food.

Peace Is Every Step: The Path of Mindfulness in Everyday Life

Thich Nhat Hanh

A classic primer on mindfulness.

The Power of Habit: Why We Do What We Do in Life and Business

Charles Duhigg

Mindful Life Weight Loss

This book explains the anatomy (cue - routine - reward) of a habit. That is the first step to changing it.

Diet

Fat Chance: Beating the Odds Against Sugar, Processed Food, Obesity, and Disease

Robert H. Lustig, MD

Great book to understand common diets and how our food supply creates addiction and overeating.

The End of Overeating: Taking Control of the Insatiable American Appetite

David A. Kessler

Excellent research-based book about how the food industry is making us sick and addicted. Eye opening.

Food Junkies: The Truth About Food Addiction

Vera Tarman, MD with Philip Werdell

An MD examines the complex topic of food addiction.

Food Rules: An Eater's Manual

Michael Pollan

A pocket guide for how to choose real food.

Relationships

Thinking in Systems: A Primer

Donella H. Meadows

Technical book about how systems theory works. The theoretical basis of the leverage points approach.

Nature

Your Brain on Nature: The Science of Nature's Influence on Your Health, Happiness and Vitality

Eva M. Selhub, MD and Alan C. Logan ND

Jam packed with scientific research about how time spent in nature can improve your health, mood, and productivity.

For an updated list, see our website: http://weightlosswestchesterny.com/weightlossbooks.html

Blog

Mindful Life Weight Loss

http://weightlosswesterny.com/weightlossblog/

Facebook Page

https://www.facebook.com/weightlosswestchesterny

About the Author

Kim Gold is the co-creator of the Mindful Life Weight Loss program. She has studied and practiced ways of personal growth through meditative disciplines and psychology for more than 25 years. She has an M.S. in Marriage and Family Therapy, is a registered yoga teacher, and holds a black belt in Aikido. Kim's former career as a medical/scientific editor has evolved into writing and teaching about health and mindfulness. She leads Mindful Life Weight Loss groups, and teaches yoga and meditation at Still Mind Martial Arts & Yoga in White Plains, NY. In her spare time, Kim can be found rescuing animals and enjoying life as a suburban parent.

http://weightlosswestchesterny.com

https://www.facebook.com/weightlosswestchesterny

http://martialartswhiteplains.com

About Integrated Peace Arts

Integrated Peace Arts is a nonsectarian, nonprofit 501(C) (3) corporation that employs the principles common to the major world religions, profound philosophies, and psychology to help people become happier and more effective in their day-to-day lives.

Integrated Peace Arts Press publishes books that align with its mission.

http://integrated-peace-arts.org